The Identification and Treatment of Trauma in Individuals with Developmental Disabilities

Sharon McGilvery, Ph.D.

Copyright © 2018 NADD Press

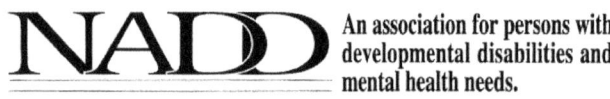 An association for persons with developmental disabilities and mental health needs.

132 Fair Street
Kingston, New York 12401

All rights reserved.

No part of this book may be reproduced, stored in a retrieval system or transmitted in any form by means of electronic, mechanical, photocopy, recording or otherwise, without written permission of NADD, 132 Fair Street, Kingston, New York 12401.

ISBN: 978-1-57256-124-3
LCCN: 2018964363

Printed in the United States of America

This book is dedicated to my father and mother, Benjamin and Sadie McGilvery, who left this world too soon. Thank you for my life, the years of kindness, your humor, and unconditional love. Until we meet again...

Table of Contents

Acknowledgements ix
Introduction xi
Chapter 1 – Definition of Trauma 1
   Trauma among individuals with intellectual disabilities................. 2
   Vulnerability to trauma and PTSD 4
Types of trauma.. 6
      The disability itself.. 7
      Sexual trauma 8
      Dysfunctional childhoods 8
      Foster care.. 8
      Uncomplicated, complicated, and traumatic grief 9
      Loss of a job 12
      Loss of family home and change of residences 12
      Institutionalized living 13
      Restraint use/aversive techniques 14
      Bullying and teasing 14
      Medical procedures and medical hospitalizations 14
      Changes in physical health 15
      Use of psychotropic medications.. 15
Chapter 2 – Impact of Trauma on the Brain 17
   Emotional regulation and emotional dysregulation..................... 20
   Executive functioning skills and deficits....................................... 22
   Emotional regulation skills training 23
   Developmental trauma 23
Chapter 3 -Diagnosis of PTSD and Trauma Based Reactions in Individuals With Developmental Disabilities 25
   Historical references to PTSD 25
   The Diagnostic and Statistical Manuals 26
      DSM-I 26
      DSM-II 26

    DSM-III 26
    DSM-III-R 27
    DSM-IV 28
    DSM-IV-TR 28
    DSM-5 29
  The Diagnostic Manual-Intellectual Disability and the DM-ID-2 30
    DM-ID-2 31
  Signs and symptoms of PTSD in individuals
    with intellectual disabilities and diagnostic complications 32
  Sub-threshold PTSD 36
  Assessing for co-morbidity 38
    PTSD and somatic symptoms 39
    Psychosis and PTSD 40

**Chapter 4 – The Identification of Trauma: Methods of Assessment
in Individuals with Intellectual Disabilities** 43
  Challenges in assessment 43
  Assessment measures 44
    PTSD symptoms and symptom severity scales 44
    Trauma exposure measures 44
    Assessment of PTSD in children 46
  Assessment of traumatic events and traumatic exposure
  for individuals with ID 46
  Possible trauma related or trauma induced behaviors 53
    Avoidance behaviors 53
    Alterations in arousal and reactivity 53
    Marked alterations in cognitive and mood 54
    Intrusive symptoms 54
  History taking and getting to know the individual 55

Chapter 5 – Trauma-Informed Treatment and Trauma-Informed Care 57
  Specific trainings in trauma sensitive interventions 60
    Strategies for administrators and managers of adult
    residential facilities 60
    Strategies for group home or adult residential facility staff 65
    Strategies for parents 67
  Care for the caretaker 68
    Care provider stress and burnout 70
    Self-care plans 71
  Trauma informed systems 74

Chapter 6 – Risks and Resiliency 77
  Pre-traumatic factors 78
  Peri-traumatic factors 79
  Post-traumatic factors 79

Predictor variables for PTSD among individuals
　　　　with intellectual disabilities 80
　Resiliency 80
　　　Promoting resiliency from trauma and stressful events
　　　　among individuals with intellectual disabilities 81
　　　Neuroplasticity and PTSD and recovery 83
Chapter 7 - Treatment of Traumatic Reactions in Individuals with ID 85
　Being safe with oneself 86
　Physical safety 86
　Feeling safe with others 87
　Specific therapies for the treatment of PTSD 88
　PTSD treatment approaches for individuals with
　　intellectual disabilities 89
　　　Eye Movement Desensitization Reprocessing (EMDR) 90
　　　Cognitive Behavioral TherapyCognitive Behavioral Therapy (CBT) . 92
　　　Stress Inoculation Training (SIT) 93
　　　Dialectical Behavior Therapy (DBT) 94
　　　Mindfulness 95
　　　Meditation 96
　　　Psychodynamic Psychotherapy 97
　　　Neurofeedback 97
　　　Yoga 98
　　　Relaxation Response Training 99
　　　Exposure Therapy 99
　　　Sensory Modulation Strategies 100
　　　Emotional Regulation Skills Training 102
　　　Animal Assisted Therapy 105
　　　Assertiveness Training 106
　　　Music Therapy 107
　　　Pharmacological Interventions 107
　Basic supportive approaches for managing trauma based
　　reactions among individuals with intellectual disabilities 108
　Interventions for specific trauma based or stress induced behaviors 112
　　　Sleep disturbances 112
　　　Anger outbursts 115
　　　Aggression 117
　Medical trauma – fearfulness with medical examinations
　　and procedures 119
　Family Environment and social support 122

Chapter 8 – Individual Stores/Case Studies 123
   How to incorporate a trauma sensitive approach into
   an analysis of behaviors 124
      Step 1: Identify the challenging behavior 125
      Step 2: Identify the type and cause of the
      developmental disability 125
      Step 3: Developmental history/ACEs 126
      Step 4: Past and present psychiatric diagnosis 126
      Step 5: Psychotropic medications 126
      Step 6: Medical conditions past and present 126
      Step 7: Placement history 126
      Step 8: Timeline of events 127
      Step 9: Changes in functioning 127
      Step 10: Current environment 127
      The final analysis 127
   John's story 128
      The analysis 129
      The final analysis-putting it all together 134
      Interventions 136
   Michael's story 139
      The analysis 140
      The final analysis 143
      Interventions 143
   David's story 144
      The analysis 145
      The final analysis 147
      Interventions 147
   Case Reflections 148
Chapter 9- A Summary 151
   The future 154
References 157
Index 173

Acknowledgements

I would like to thank Kimberly Gaines-Williams, Ph.D., and Katie Taylor Gerran, LMFT, for their feedback and their dedication to this field. Their hard work and their day-to-day resolve to help this population are inspirational. I would also like to acknowledge the rest of my colleagues at the San Diego Regional Center: Michael Raulston, Christie Torge, Leah Wall, Zeltzin Munoz, Randy Deleon, Erik Peterson, and Erin Rodriquez. They have to confront the frustrations and complexities of systems, legalities, budgetary constraints, limited resources, client and care provider traumas, and they must do so all in a day's work. My appreciation and thanks also extend to Becky Wergers, RN, for her unwavering dedication to the clients we serve.

At Inland Regional Center, thanks extend to Mary Pounders, MA, Program Manager, for the cases she has given me which served as an impetus for this book and for her years of professional dedication to this field. I would also like to express my gratitude to my colleague, Barbara Begley, MSW, who has worked with me side by side on some very difficult cases involving trauma during the past few years.

Finally, a special thanks to my husband, Alden Merrill, who not only helped make it possible for me to spend hours writing this book but helped me tackle the technology gremlins frequently lurking in my computer.

Introduction

This book was born out of necessity. I intend it as a resource for differing audiences ranging from novice care providers to seasoned practitioners who have not yet recognized the pivotal role of trauma in the behaviors of the clients they serve. Recognizing the influence of trauma in the assessment of behaviors of individuals with intellectual disabilities, and trauma's role in the development of effective interventions, adds a crucial additional dimension to our understanding of an often misunderstood population. Both assessing and treating trauma must be foremost in the consciousness of clinicians as well as daily care providers.

As a behavioral consultant for the past several decades, I commonly receive referrals on individuals whose behavioral reputations are severe. They are typically well known to local psychiatric hospitals, the local police, and sundry institutions and agencies. Often their families are distraught trying to manage difficult behavioral challenges without fully understanding why the behaviors occur and what they could do to help. Residential staff members have difficulty managing the behaviors of individuals dwelling in community facilities or residences. The individuals themselves often have lengthy histories of failed placements, accompanied by dispiriting lists of psychiatric diagnoses and sometimes longer lists of medications. As I began to work with these individuals, I realized that their complex histories often included many different forms of trauma and stress. It was not until I fully appreciated the impact these events had in their lives that I was able to create interventions which were more effective. It is truly said that, "Necessity is the mother of invention." I needed to learn or devise other routes of intervention to address some of the behavioral challenges stemming from past traumas that were manifesting in the present. As I integrated patients' trauma histories with contemporary research in the area of trauma, I was able to incorporate trauma-informed strategies and approaches into my behavioral plans.

Little in the psychological literature addressed trauma assessment in individuals with intellectual disabilities. Thus, I devised my own questionnaires for families and staff to use as a reference for reviewing case histories. I also learned specific questions to ask individuals to elicit first-hand information regarding their experiences. This too was demanded by necessity, because there is a lack of standardized assessment measures for assessing for posttraumatic stress disorder (PTSD) or subclinical symptoms of PTSD in this population. Consequently, the questionnaires I developed were derived from experiences acquired in the metaphorical trenches of behavioral consulting. Accomplishing this required sensitivity to the great variety of trauma and stress that individuals with intellectual disabilities may encounter in their lives. These events encompass a broad range of experiences. I also learned to judge their reactions by their standards and perceptions and not by mine. What one person may find stressful or traumatic, another may not. Such individual variability must be considered and anticipated when working in this area.

Beginning in the assessment phase, I had to learn how to view certain behavioral challenges as possible reflections of the trauma they experienced. This included being sensitive to the physical changes that can occur in the brain with trauma and to the behaviors that may be symptomatic of trauma-based reactions. This path indicated the types of treatment approaches that should be the most effective. Among all the treatment approaches I researched, certain core concepts emerged that were prominent and critical. These included the need to re-establish safety, consistency, predictability, choice, and control. Whatever specific treatments were used, such as cognitive-behavioral or exposure treatments, basic elements needed to be established in order to promote healing. After these realizations, I learned that some of the most effective approaches I used were those which incorporated strategies to decrease physical and emotional arousal among those individuals with severe emotional and behavioral challenges. Teaching techniques to self-soothe, calm down, lower reactivity, and manage anger and anxiety were some of the most helpful techniques. This book includes case studies that reflect many of these interventions. The need to focus on improving self-regulation skills, as well as the need to incorporate positive experiences and remove trauma triggers, also prompted staff trainings and trainings for family members on these constructs. These concepts are also discussed in this book.

My journey of discovery also led to a review of the psychological literature. I found a plethora of findings and research on PTSD and its treatment among the general population. However, there was a dearth of related literature and research involving individuals with intellectual disabilities, certainly in comparison with related publications concerning the general population. There is a notable paucity of systematic and controlled studies on the efficacy of different therapeutic approaches in treating trauma affecting individuals with intellectual disabilities.

This book, essentially, follows a timeline of the path that I had to take from an appreciation of the different types of trauma, to its identification in a much underserved population, to the identification of meaningful interventions, and to the training of support personnel. The chapters often begin with the findings of the research in the general population and then proceed to the extrapolation and application of some of these findings to this special population.

The complexity of trauma among this population requires a thorough understanding of trauma, its roots, and its impact and an appreciation of the need for trauma-informed care and approaches. Much research is still needed in the area, as individuals with intellectual disabilities continue to be an underserved and often misunderstood population.

Chapter 1

Trauma Defined

"The world breaks everyone, and afterward, many are strong at the broken places."
  – Ernest Hemingway

Traumatic events occur as part of life and part of the human condition. Sometimes traumatizing experiences occur for reasons that are beyond our control, as in the case of natural disasters such as hurricanes or floods. Sometimes traumatic events occur due to human error, ignorance, or negligence, or even deliberately at the hands of others. Horrific situations can also occur when badly timed circumstances or accidental events combine with a catastrophic result. The definition of trauma can be broad and encompass many different types of incidents and experiences.

Ozer and Weiss (2004) reported that 50% to 90% of the adult population will experience a traumatic event in their lifetimes. According to the Substance Abuse and Mental Health Services Administration (SAMHSA, 2014), "In the United States, 61% of men and 51 % of women report exposure to at least one lifetime traumatic event, and 90% of clients in public health care settings have experienced trauma." There is a higher prevalence rate of trauma among individuals who are being served by a variety of social service systems. According to researchers (Adams, 2010; Sprague, 2008), 75% - 93% of youth who have entered the juvenile justice system have experienced traumatic victimization. According to the National Center for Children in Poverty (Cooper, 2007), 50% of children who have been involved in the child welfare system have suffered from trauma. Some studies have shown a high rate of trauma in the histories of individuals seeking services for substance abuse (Jennings, 2004). Researchers have also found that a majority of individuals admitted to inpatient psychiatric facilities have experienced various forms of trauma in their pasts (van der Kolk, 1996).

So why focus on trauma if it is an inevitable part of the human condition? Because ongoing research has shown that its impact can be pervasive and potentially life altering. It can predispose people to a variety of psychiatric conditions as well as physical illnesses (SAMHSA, 2014). It can adversely impact and negatively transform relationships. If the results of the trauma are debilitating enough, it can lead to a diagnosis of posttraumatic stress disorder or to other psychiatric conditions which can interfere with an individual's growth and day-to-day functioning (SAMHSA, 2014). If the consequences of trauma remain unaddressed, they can render interventions ineffective for mental health conditions, and they can result in poorer health outcomes.

The pervasive impact of trauma really came to light in a landmark study that was the result of a collaboration between the Center for Disease Control (CDC) and Kaiser Permanente (1998). It explored the impact early traumatic experiences can have on the health of individuals spanning into adulthood. The pioneering study was referred to as the Adverse Childhood Experiences Study (ACE Study), and it was one of largest studies conducted. It included 17,000 participants from Southern California who were recruited from 1995 to 1997. Participants were involved in long-term follow-up assessments to examine physical health outcomes. They were asked to complete confidential surveys regarding their experiences as children and their current health conditions. Researchers found strong associations between early childhood adverse experiences and physical, social, and behavioral problems throughout the participants' lifespans. The adverse childhood experiences included physical and sexual abuse, as well as stress from parental separation or divorce and mental illness among parents. They found that individuals with adverse childhood experiences were at an increased risk for diseases such as cancer, heart disease, chronic obstructive pulmonary disease, obesity, and liver disease. In addition, there were increased risks for drug and alcohol abuse, depression, and suicide attempts. Researchers also found a dose-response relationship between the number of adverse childhood experiences and health problems. This ACE Study served as an impetus for further examining the impact early trauma can have on an individual's mental and physical well-being. It helped to lay the foundation for the concept of trauma-informed care.

There are a wide variety of events which can be considered traumatic in addition to adverse early childhood experiences which can elicit trauma-based reactions. Individual trauma results when an individual experiences certain events or circumstances which are either physically or emotionally threatening. These experiences can overwhelm an individual's ability to cope and can adversely impact his or her mental health, as well the person's spiritual and physical health (SAMHSA, 2014). When the experiences overwhelm the individual's coping mechanism to the extent that they significantly impair the individual's ability to function, it may warrant a diagnosis of posttraumatic stress disorder. However, there is also some individual variability in how people interpret, respond to, and process these events, and not everyone who experiences a traumatic event develops posttraumatic stress disorder. Some researchers, such as Russell and Shab (2003), estimate that 25% of individuals who are exposed to trauma develop PTSD. Consequently, there are other factors other than simply being exposed to a traumatic event that contribute to the development of PTSD.

What may be a traumatic event for one individual may not necessarily constitute a traumatic event for another individual, but there are some definite sources of agreement or commonalities. It is important, however, to be sensitive to the wide variety and types of trauma that can impact someone's life and the individual variability that can be present in evaluating its effects.

Trauma in Individuals with Intellectual Disabilities

An understanding of trauma and its treatment is particularly important given the reported prevalence rates of abuse among individuals with intellectual disabilities. There has been little research and little training regarding how abuse and its impact should transform care among this population. This shortage of training and research has occurred despite statistics which reveal higher rates of certain types of abuse among this population. Given some of the vulnerabilities of this population, the high prevalence rate of abuse among them, and the possibility of underreporting, it is important to learn and recognize their symptoms of trauma. According to James (1989) and Valenti-Hein and Schwartz (1995), it is estimated that only 1 in 30 instances of sexual abuse are reported among individuals with developmental disabilities. This is in stark contrast to their findings of 1 in 5 cases being reported for the general population. The greater the severity of the disability, the greater the likelihood that the individual will be abused (Sobsey, 1994). Valenti-Hein and Swartz found that individuals with developmental disabilities experience 2.5 to 10 times the abuse and neglect as compared to their non-disabled peers. More than 90% of adults with disabilities reported sexual abuse within their lifetime with 49% of that sample reporting 10 or more abusive incidents. It is interesting to note that Kendall-Tackett (2002) reported that individuals who have more than one disability are at a higher risk for both physical and sexual abuse.

In a study by Sullivan (2009), who reviewed 50 articles which were published during an eight year period from 2000 to 2008, it was found that sufficient research existed indicating that children and youth with disabilities were in a greater risk category to become victims of violence. These findings were consistent across studies which were conducted in a variety of social service settings to include child welfare agencies, health care, educational settings, and law enforcement. This was also noted to be the case internationally as the research also examined cases in Canada, Great Britain, Norway, Australia, and Israel, as well as the United States.

According to the U.S. Department of Justice, Office of Justice Programs, between 2011 and 2015, approximately 60 out of 1000 individuals, who were 12 and older and had a cognitive disability, were reportedly the victims of violence. From 2009-2011, there was an annual average of 923,000 nonfatal crimes committed against individuals with disabilities age 12 or older (Harrell, 2017). Nonfatal crimes included violent victimization such as rape, sexual assaultive, robbery, and aggravated and simple assault. (Disabilities are classified in these statistics according to the following limitations: cognitive, sensory, self-care, ambulation, and independent living.) During the period from 2009 – 2011, statistics from the U.S. Department of Justice referencing self-reported victims of abuse noted that 62% had an intellectual disability and 66.5% had autism. Statistics varied by disability. For those with an intellectual or developmental disability, 43.2 % reported sexual abuse. The following are U.S. Department of Justice 2011 age-adjusted rates of violent victimization rates per 1,000 (Harrell, 2017):

	People with Disabilities	*People without Disabilities*
Rape/sexual assault	2.7	0.9
Robbery	8.3	1.8
Aggravated assault	10.6	3.3
Simple assault	26.1	13.4
Males	42	22
Females	53	17

According to statistics provided by U.S. Department of Justice in 2011, only 37.3% of individuals with disabilities who were the victims of abuse reported their abuse to the authorities. The Department also found that, "...when families of victims and people with disabilities who are victims are both considered, the rate of reporting increased to 51.7%. This suggests that when a family member learns of abuse, it becomes more likely that a report will be filed with authorities."

The U.S. Department of Justice also reported statistics regarding what transpired after reports of abuse were made to authorities. In 52.5% of the cases that were reported, nothing occurred as a result of the reporting. In 9.8% of the cases, the individual who committed the crime was arrested. The statistics changed when the incidents were reported by both the families and the victim with disabilities. In those cases, 42.8% of the reports resulted in nothing happening, and the percent of alleged perpetrators who were arrested decreased to 7.8%.

The following are statistics from the U.S. Department of Justice reports for 2011 for bullying (reported by people with disabilities and families): 77% for individuals with autism and 64.3% for individuals with intellectual disabilities. The following are the statistics provided by the Department with regard to the frequency of receiving therapy and the frequency of abuse:

- 65.4% of individuals who were the victims of abuse or bullying did not receive any counseling or therapy.
- More than 63% of individuals who were the victims of physical abuse did not receive therapy.
- 52% of sexual assault victims did not receive therapy.
- In the cases in which therapy was provided, 83% of people with disabilities believed it was helpful.
- With regard to the frequency of abuse, more than 90% of people with disabilities who reported that abuse occurred stated it occurred on multiples occasions. Fifty-seven percent of these victims claimed they had been the victims of abuse on more than 20 occasions with 46% reporting that it had happened with so much frequency that it was difficult to provide an accurate number.

In addition to being exposed to greater risks of being physically and/or sexually abused, researchers have also found children with intellectual disabilities tend to experience a greater number of negative life events. Such events have included changes in residence, bereavement, life-threatening illnesses, and interpersonal conflicts, etc. (Hatton & Emerson, 2004). It has also been suggested by researchers that the range of potentially traumatic events among individuals with intellectual disabilities is larger than those in the general population (Martorell & Tsakanikos, 2008).

Vulnerability to Trauma and PTSD

Given the prevalence rate of abuse among individuals with intellectual disabilities, coupled with a higher rate of psychiatric disorders as compared to the general population, it becomes critical to monitor for trauma-based reactions. Individuals with developmental disabilities are at an increased risk for the development of all psychiatric conditions including posttraumatic stress disorder with figures estimated to be three to four times the prevalence rates found among the general population (Cooper,

Smiley, Morrison, Williamson, & Allan, 2007). This existing vulnerability for psychiatric disorders, coupled with a higher risk of abuse, can elevate the risk of developing PTSD or trauma-based reactions.

What makes this population more vulnerable to various forms of abuse and traumatic experiences? There are a variety of factors, including the following:

1. *Level of expressive language skills* – At the lower levels of cognitive functioning, the individual is usually non-verbal. This can also be one of the reasons why they are at a greater risk to be abused because they are not able to speak about the abuse or to notify someone.
2. *Dependence on caretakers* – As some individuals with intellectual disabilities are dependent upon caretakers to help them meet their day-to-day needs, they become potentially more vulnerable to abuse, or other forms of trauma, from the very people charged with their care. As their level of care increases, it can also set the stage for greater dependency upon the very individuals who may have injured them, either physically or emotionally.
3. *Stress on caretakers* – The high level of stress sometimes experienced by family members or other care providers can make the individual with an intellectual disability more vulnerable to abuse. High levels of stress can also lead to more family conflicts. Family members who also provide care on an ongoing basis can become exhausted and experience "burn out."
4. *Lack of credibility* – This can be particularly problematic for individuals who are higher functioning and who frequently may make false allegations against their caretakers. Although there are regulations governing how allegations of abuse are handled in community residences or institutions, an investigation may be only perfunctory, and the individual's allegations can be too quickly dismissed. A person may not be perceived as a credible reporter due to his or her disability. Because of a history of behavioral challenges that include false allegations against care providers, actual incidents of abuse may not be thoroughly explored and may be quickly dismissed.
5. *Physical limitations* – The physical limitations of the individual can affect their ability to communicate abuse or leave situations.
6. *Low Self Esteem* – Williams and Poijula (2002) posit that self-esteem can help an individual cope with abuse. Self-esteem is built and reinforced by many factors. These can include not only the mastery of certain activities but also receiving praise and positive feedback. Individuals with intellectual disabilities may have heard more about their weaknesses and skill deficits rather than their strengths and may suffer from insufficient opportunities to experience success. Consequently, they may not have the confidence to speak up, or they may not believe they deserve better treatment.
7. *Cognitive limitations* – An individual's cognitive limitations may make it difficult for the person to identify high risk situations for abuse and avoid them. A cognitive disability could also limit the individual's ability to comprehend what is happening in a situation or what is being asked of them. The person may agree to what is being asked while not fully comprehending the seriousness of the violation.
8. *Need to fit in* – The person may also want to fit in and, therefore, may be vulnerable to manipulation. For example, if someone with a mild to moderate

intellectual disability has a strong desire to fit in, that individual may be more easily persuaded into engaging in gang-related activity or drug dealing activities without fully comprehending the potential consequences.
9. *Limited opportunities to develop friendships/relationships* – Individuals with intellectual disabilities often lack the opportunities to develop friendships. Consequently, their support systems may be very limited. If so, individuals may be more likely to want to please or gain the approval and attention of others. This may make them more likely to accept abuse or tolerate mistreatment.
10. *Compliance to authority figures* –Valenti-Hein and Swartz (1995) proposed that increased vulnerability for abuse among individuals with developmental disabilities may be attributed to the fact that some have been taught to be compliant with people in authority. Although this can be said of the general population as well, we are also taught to question and to be aware of certain dangers or warning signs given by even those in authority.
11. *Lack of training or education* – The individual may not have received any formalized training in creating healthy boundaries and in sex education. They may not have an understanding of what constitutes abuse and how to be an effective advocate for themselves.

TYPES OF TRAUMA

A traumatic event can cause psychological trauma when it overwhelms the individual's ability to cope. The individual may experience a single event or a series of events. Trauma can occur in many different forms with the more common ones consisting of sexual or physical abuse. However, in supporting individuals with intellectual disabilities it is important to be aware of the many potential sources of trauma including the disability itself. The following is a list of some possible sources of trauma and stress for individuals with intellectual disabilities:
- The disability itself
- Dysfunctional childhoods characterized by living in chaotic and highly conflicted environments, childhood neglect
- Emotional abuse
- Physical abuse
- Sexual abuse
- Trauma from institutionalized living
- Trauma from any situation which creates a sense of powerlessness
- Threats of loss of attachments
- Losses of property
- Encounters with law enforcement
- The use of restrictive interventions such as physical restraints
- Being forced to take medications and experiencing adverse or frightening side effects
- Bullying
- Teasing
- Social rejection
- Invasive medical procedures and/or medical hospitalizations

- Significant changes in physical health, including accidental physical injury
- Psychiatric hospitalizations
- Social neglect
- Impaired care providers (e.g., caregiver depression, substance abuse, or caregiver medical illness)
- The cumulative effect of a series of adverse experiences
- Loss of relationships including family, staff, and peers
- Changes in living arrangements
- Peer conflicts
- Separations from parents
- Receiving a discharge notice from a residential placements
- Loss of a job
- Sexual harassment
- Threat of physical violence
- Living in congregate living arrangements with aggressive peers or peers with other challenging behaviors
- Sexual abuse and physical abuse by peers
- Threats of loss
- Threats of out-of-home placement
- Victim of violent crime
- Witnessing domestic violence

This proposed list is by no means an all-inclusive one. In considering the different types of trauma, it is also important to consider what Shapiro (2001) has labeled as the concept of the small "t" trauma. These can consist of adverse life experiences or a series of upsetting events that may not constitute life threatening or major events, but they can still do damage (Marich, 2014). The cumulative effect of small stressful events also has the capability of adversely impacting one's physical as well as mental health (Esbensen & Benson, 2006).

The Disability Itself

Of the potential sources of trauma that have been identified, sometimes one of the most difficult for individuals to grapple with is the diagnosis of having a disability. Coming to grips with the reality that one has a disability and is different from the rest can be traumatizing in and of itself (Levitas & Gibson, 2001). Historically, an intellectual disability was termed "mental retardation." To hear that term applied to oneself can be very distressing and even traumatic. Gentile and Gillig (2012) discussed "ordinary" life event trauma which may include not only feeling different because of the disability but also feeling ignored, feeling misunderstood, not having the opportunities, or not having the ability to do what others are doing. Moreover, it has been suggested that viewing oneself as being disabled is potentially traumatizing. It is another factor that may contribute to an elevated risk of developing PTSD (Levitas & Gibson, 2001). The disability itself and the stigma attached to it, as well as the cumulative experiences the individual has encountered throughout the years as a result of the disability, can be traumatic.

Sexual Trauma

In the general population, a history of sexual abuse has been associated with PTSD as well as a variety of other psychiatric conditions including depression, anxiety disorders, mood disorders, medical conditions, eating disorders, substance abuse, and personality disorders (van der Kolk, 1996). Among individuals with intellectual disabilities, a history of sexual abuse has also been found to be associated with higher rates of anxiety, depression, and sexually inappropriate behaviors including promiscuity, avoidance, or a preoccupation with sex (Matich-Maroney, 2003).

Dysfunctional Childhoods

The topic of childhood abuse and neglect as a form of trauma deserves particular attention due to the high rate of potentially negative outcomes it can have, not only in the general population, but among individuals with developmental disabilities. The risks of adverse childhood experiences (ACEs) are greater in children with disabilities. According to Sullivan and Knutson (2000), there is a 3.76 times greater risk of neglect, a 3.79 times greater risk of physical abuse, and 3.14 times greater risk of sexual abuse.

If a child has experienced multiple traumas (i.e., complex trauma), it can also impact the child's developmental trajectory in a variety of ways. It can lead to multiple psychiatric diagnoses, developmental impairments, and numerous behavioral issues. Therefore, it is important to complete a thorough assessment that also includes the identification of various traumatic events that may be associated with developmental delays or derailments.

Foster Care

Of special mention are individuals with intellectual disabilities who have been placed in the foster care system at a young age due to traumatic family histories. Often, they are not only separated from their families but separated quickly to ensure their physical safety. Consequently, the child may have experienced multiple traumas. First, they are quickly separated from their parents and placed in new homes with individuals they do not know, or admitted to a facility for children, until a foster placement can be located. This may be followed by a series of other foster homes. If the child's behaviors become too difficult to manage, or the behaviors present a danger, the child may either be psychiatrically hospitalized or admitted to a group home. Consequently, there may be multiples disruptions in the child's attachment history. According to United Cerebral Palsy Association (2006), there were more than half a million children and youth who were placed in the foster care system in the United States. Among those children, studies indicated that approximately one-third had disabilities and those disabilities ranged from mild intellectual delays to significant physical disabilities and psychiatric disabilities (Vig, Chinitz, & Shulman, 2005).

Looking at statistics from the general population, some studies have suggested that between 19.2% and 21% of foster care alumni suffer from symptoms of PTSD which is a rate higher than the statistics for United States veterans of war (Kolko et al., 2010; Pecora et al., 2005). Although studies are lacking which have explored the prevalence rate of PTSD symptoms, or even sub-threshold PTSD symptoms, in individuals with intellectual disabilities who have been in foster care, the statistics obtained from the general population are disconcerting. The implications of these statistics for an even more vulnerable population of individuals with intellectual disabilities should result in a heighten monitoring and sensitivity to these issues.

Uncomplicated, Complicated, and Traumatic Grief

Of the list of potential sources of trauma, particular attention should be paid to those situations involving grief and loss. There are many potential sources of loss for individuals with intellectual disabilities. Losses can include disrupted attachment histories. Grief may also be present in response to other types of losses that occur such as a loss of a residence if the individual is forced to move. The person may have sustained losses of friendships due to having to move into different residential settings. Losses can also exist in the form of symbolic losses. Individuals with intellectual disabilities may have experienced numerous losses throughout their lifetimes with the most significant losses being the death of someone close to them.

Despite the numerous losses that individuals with intellectual disabilities may encounter, the grief process they experience is often overlooked or dismissed. This becomes especially true among those with severe or profound intellectual disabilities and may occur for several reasons. First, it may be due to confusion about how they process loss. However, as Brickell and Munir (2008) noted, "Even without a cognitive understanding of death, however, it is possible to notice the absence of a loved one and to react emotionally to that loss." Second, care providers may want to spare the person emotional pain so information may be withheld. This writer recalls one situation in which a client living in an institution was not told that his mother died. Staff was fearful that he would react poorly to the loss. Other staff, to include some family members, felt the explanation was unnecessary because they thought his cognitive level was too low for him to either understand the loss or even notice her absence. He had an intellectual disability that was in the severe range. His mother used to come faithfully for years to visit him on the weekends until she died suddenly of a heart attack. Neither his family, nor the staff, provided him with an explanation of her absence, since they questioned whether or not the loss would be really meaningful to him. However, he stopped eating several weeks after her death, and he had to be spoon fed. It was discovered later that when his mother came to visit him every weekend she would spoon feed him even though he was able to feed himself. It was her way of caring for her son.

A third reason why the grief process may be overlooked or compromised for individuals with intellectual disabilities is that well-meaning care providers or family members may not want to tell the person the whole truth at one time. Sometimes family members or staff have opted to gradually break the news to the person thinking this would be easier to accept when given in incremental truths. Although, disclosing information over time may be less upsetting and even helpful in some circumstances, it could cause further problems if the lack of disclosure limits or prevents the person from participating in family events or grieving rituals. In addition, if the individual has very challenging behaviors, care providers may not want to inform the person, or help them process the loss, out of concern or fear that the individual's behavioral challenges may significantly increase.

Research studies on the grieving process, including factors which can facilitate an adaptation to loss as well as complicate it, have been sparse for individuals with intellectual disabilities. There have been a few researchers and theorists who believe that grief reactions deserve a more focused study among vulnerable populations such as individuals with intellectual disabilities (ID). Brickell and Munir (2008) proposed that individuals with ID are more susceptible to traumatic grief based on several factors including difficulties communicating about the loss, difficulty finding meaning in the loss due to cognitive impairments and having an increased risk of secondary losses. Secondary losses are those additional losses that occur as a result of the initial loss, and they can also be traumatic. For example, if an individual with an intellectual disability lives with her mother and her mother dies suddenly, the individual may have to move into a facility or a community residence. Consequently, the individual has not only lost her mother, but she has also lost her home. Perhaps, she has also had to change day programs or jobs as a result of the death of her parent. If this were the case, consider how many losses the individual sustained as a result of her primary loss.

Brickell and Munir (2008) noted that because of these three factors (i.e., communication difficulties, secondary losses, and difficulty processing the meaning) among bereaved individuals with ID it is more difficult for them to accommodate and adapt to the loss. This can complicate the grief process and make the grief more likely to be traumatic. A traumatic grief reaction is considered to be distinct from a normal grief reaction due to a marked intensity of numerous symptoms including separation anxiety, yearning, searching, anger, and excessive irritability, etc. The symptoms persist and remain at a marked level of intensity after the loss causing significant impairment in the individual's ability to function (Horowitz et al., 1997). With traumatic grief, there is not only grief but there is a concurrent form of traumatic distress (Jacobs & Prigerson, 2000). Traumatic grief is a severe form of bereavement which shares some similarities with PTSD. It is a complicated or "pathological" form of grief in which the individual is experiencing complications adjusting to the loss and recovering effectively.

Among the general population, researchers and grief theorists have tried to identify symptoms of grief or aspects of the grieving process that can predict long-term impairment. Among those investigators, Rando (1993) spoke about complicated versus uncomplicated grief reactions. According to Rando, what helps determine the course of grief, and whether or not grief will become complicated or move towards a healthy adaptation, is whether or not the tasks of mourning have been completed. Those tasks, referred to as the "Six R Processes of Mourning" by Rando are as follows:

1. *Recognizing the loss*
2. *Reacting to the separation and loss* – This involves also processing secondary losses which are additional losses resulting from the primary loss.
3. *Recollecting and re-experiencing*
4. *Relinquishing old attachments*
5. *Readjusting-* This involves forming a new relationship with the deceased based on the physical absence of the person. Just because someone dies does not mean the individual ends that relationship. The relationship may live on in the heart and mind of the bereaved person, but it is now transformed.
6. *Reinvesting* – This occurs when the person is accommodating to the loss.

According to Rando (1993), normal mourning would involve the successful completion of all these tasks but not necessarily in the order with which they are listed. Rando also noted that individuals are more predisposed to traumatic grief if the bereaved had been dependent upon the deceased for their care. Other researchers such as Selby (1999) have found that individuals who sustain a loss, and experience that loss as traumatic, are at a higher risk for severe health difficulties as well as psychiatric issues. Finally, the trauma response and its consequences can disrupt the mourning process and perpetuate complicated grief patterns of thinking and behaving (Raphael, 1983).

For individuals with intellectual disabilities, adapting to a loss and moving forward can be complicated by a number of factors which can, in theory, exacerbate the grief process and hinder healing. Examples include the following:

- Sometimes they are not invited to the funeral when funerals can help add meaning and acceptance by confronting the realty of the loss.
- Sometimes they are deprived of the opportunity to process the loss by talking with people and working it through.
- The loss may have been more sudden to them because they were not included earlier in the process if their loved one had a terminal illness.
- Also, the grieving process may have been discouraged by well-intentioned care providers. This may result in the individual with an intellectual disability receiving little support or assistance in processing the loss and adapting to the new situation. As Wadsworth and Harper (1991) noted, if an individual with an intellectual disability is unprepared for dealing with the loss, and receives little or no support, this could result in long-standing behavioral problems and emotional issues. The individual may be non-verbal and lack a formal way to communicate reactions to the loss which can further complicate the situation.

Unfortunately, studies of bereavement and the factors that facilitate healing among individuals with ID have been lacking. In an early study conducted by Emerson (1977) of grief among individuals with an intellectual disability, it was found that in half the cases they reviewed, in which new behavioral challenges emerged (including physical and/or verbal aggression and social withdrawal), individuals had experienced a loss or death of someone close. Hollins and Kloeppel (1989) conducted one of the earliest studies of bereavement among individuals with intellectual disabilities. In their study, 50 grieving adults with ID were matched for age and disability against 50 controls. Several measures were used including the Aberrant Behavior Checklist and the Psychopathology Instrument for Mentally Retarded Adults. The study found that the bereaved group had significantly more cases of depression and anxiety disorders than the matched control group. Also, the bereaved group participants were more hyperactive, irritable, and lethargic.

To date, there has been little research or consideration given to identifying the differences between normal or healthy grief and pathological grief (to include traumatic grief reactions) among individuals with intellectual disabilities. Brickell and Munir (2008) believe this may be due to the concept referred to as "diagnostic overshadowing." This occurs when an individual's responses are attributed to his or her developmental disability. The disability overshadows other considerations and the person's behaviors or emotional reactions are attributed to the disability itself. However, identifying traumatic grief reactions and complicated grief in individuals with intellectual disabilities has the potential to improve their clinical care and ensure proper emotional supports. There may also be a tendency to minimize or not appreciate the losses incurred by an individual with an intellectual disability due to language deficits and cognitive impairments. The loss may not even fit into the category of "traumatic grief" as the term has been defined by some researchers among the general population, but it may nonetheless have been traumatizing to the individual and should not be disregarded.

Loss of a Job

The loss of a job or loss of a day program can also be trauma producing. For an individual with an intellectual disability, being fired from a job can be very stressful (as it can for anyone in the general population). However, since paying jobs may be more difficult to secure for someone with a developmental disability, the impact of the loss may be even greater. I am reminded of the man with autism and a mild intellectual disability who was working at a job for several months. He was working on an assembly line, and he had a job coach to help support his efforts. After six months of being the most productive worker on site, he was fired for commenting on the secretary's new dress. He stated, "You look as good as a piece of cake." He was fired for sexual harassment. While talking to him about his experience and trying to help him make sense of the loss, he said, "Why do people tell me to watch what I say when their words cut my throat?" When asked to explain his statement, he said he had overheard some of the staff saying that it wasn't a real job anyway. His losses in this circumstance were compounded not only being terminated from the job, but also by his feeling that his work efforts were being demeaned (not to mention that his attempts at complimenting a co-worker were misunderstood).

Loss of Family Home and Change of Residences

Obtaining information about an individual's residential history is important and can provide clues to the existence of any trauma-based reactions. For example, when did the individual leave the family home? How old was the person at the time, and what does the individual remember about the circumstances? What was his or her understanding of the move? How many other places had the individual lived and what reactions and behaviors occurred after the move?

After speaking with many individuals with developmental disabilities throughout the years, I have heard numerous stories from them about their memories of being taken away from their family home. Some families requested out-of-home placement out of desperation because they were unable to manage the individual's behavioral challenges or medical needs. Some were removed from their family homes for their own safety by Child Protective Services as a result of parental abuse and neglect. In either scenario, I am always struck by how many adults have an ultimate goal to return home to be with their family of origin even after many years of living apart. Some also struggle with messages they received early on with regard to the reason why they had to leave their home. One young man in his 20's told me that he was told by a social worker that his family didn't love him anymore. Whether or not that was actual the message he received is unknown, but it was his memory or perception of it that was important.

Some individuals have had to leave community residences, foster homes, or group homes through no fault of their own. The care provider may have decided to retire, or the individuals' medical needs exceeded the level of support the care provider could provide. Some were asked to leave because of their behavioral challenges and due to dangers they may have presented to the staff or other residents. Some may have received discharge notices after being admitted to a psychiatric facility and were never given an opportunity to say good-bye or obtain any type of closure. Friendships that they may have developed in that home may have ended abruptly with no further contact between them and their peers or care providers. Understandably, there are times when living in a particular setting may not meet an individual's needs or may present an unsafe situation for care providers and other residents. However, it can still be very difficult to process and absorb so many changes so quickly, not to mention the impact that it may have on an individual's self-esteem. Sometimes the individual is not quite sure of the reasons for the move and no explanation may have been provided.

Institutionalized Living

For a small number of the population with intellectual disabilities, state institutions have been their home if they had significant behavioral challenges, or complicated health care needs, which could not be supported in the community. Admissions to such state-run institutions are usually mandated by court order. Under these circumstances, the individual did not have a say in where they were going to live, nor the limits it would impose on their personal liberties. In addition, individuals who have had to live in such congregate settings may have had to reside with other residents who exhibited significant behavioral issues. Some of these behaviors may have been very frightening and threatening to others such as physical aggression, emotional outbursts, and/or verbal threats. Living with individuals who exhibit these behaviors can leave an individual feeling insecure, anxious, or worried. The person may have witnessed others becoming violent and having to be physically restrained for safety reasons. They may have also been the victims of assaults. Such situations can create a sense of powerlessness and fear. Consequently, understanding the types of living arrangement an individual has experienced may also help make sense of some of the current behaviors being displayed. For example, I am reminded of an individual who lived in an institution on another coast for years as an adolescent. Upon his relocation to another facility in another state, he would engage in pica which is the eating of inedible objects. This necessitated trips to the hospital to prevent intestinal obstruction, and in some instances he required surgery resulting in a longer stay. A review of his history referenced incidents of abuse of the residents in his original facility and the facility was eventually closed. He began eating inedible objects as a way to escape abuse by the staff because it would result in him being sent out of the facility for medical attention. This would allow him to have a temporary reprieve from the abuse and trauma in his environment.

Restraint Use/Aversive Techniques

Restraints have a long history of use in psychiatric facilities and state developmental facilities when individuals have not been responsive to other methods of calming down and they have posed a significant physical danger to others. Restraint usage could involve a variety of techniques. A manual restraint may involve staff physically holding the person down until calm, or it can involve the use of mechanical restraints such as straps that could restrict an individual's freedom of movement. Restraint devices may also include arm restraints, wrist-to-waist restraints, or hand mitts. Many years ago, seclusion rooms were also used in some state developmental centers in response to a resident's aggressive behavior or severe property destruction. Although the use of some of the more restrictive devices and techniques have been discontinued in many facilities, the individual with an intellectual disability may have been exposed to their use if he or she has had a history of institutionalized living and aggressive or self-injurious behaviors.

Despite the use of restraints in some state facilities or psychiatric facilities for individuals with intellectual disabilities over the years, there is a lack of studies which have examined the psychological impact their use may have on this population. However, it is still important to remain sensitive to the individual's history and whether or not restraint use was part of his or her experience. It is possible that a history of restraint use may have produced feelings of confusion, helplessness, and fear. It is possible that individuals with lower levels of intellectual functioning (within the severe and profound range) may have had even greater adverse emotional reactions as a result.

Bullying and Teasing

This type of abuse is sometimes referred to as "non-contact" abuse (McCreary & Thompson, 1999). Individuals with developmental disabilities are sometimes teased and called names because they are cognitively slower or grouped into another category from their peers while in school. This author has heard many individuals with intellectual disabilities discuss their anger at being called "stupid" or "slow." These experiences can contribute to low self-esteem, humiliation, a sense of outrage, and sometimes result in social withdrawal. Individuals who have experienced such taunting from their peers or others may refuse to return to the site of those mockings, thereby narrowing their opportunities and experiences in the world. It is interesting to note that there is a body of research on the neuroscience of social pain which may also apply to individuals with ID. Neuroscientists have found that social pain can occur from situations such as bullying, being taunted, being teased, or being rejected. This activates the same areas of the brain that are activated when someone is in physical pain. According to Novembre, Zanon, and Silani (2014), "Our data have shown that in conditions of social pain there is activation of an area traditionally associated with the sensory processing of physical pain, the posterior insular cortex." Therefore, being bullied or rejected or experiencing other forms of social pain can physically hurt.

Medical Procedures and Medical Hospitalizations

Even for the bravest among us, the thought of, or experience with invasive, medical procedures may be anxiety provoking. Being hospitalized and then suddenly placed in a new environment with new people can be disorienting and frightening to individuals with intellectual disabilities. The experience of pain associated with medical procedures and the experience of sedating medications can also contribute to intense emotional trauma.

Changes in Physical Health

A significant change in an individual's physical health can result in traumatic stress symptoms. For example, consider an individual who goes in for surgery to correct a spinal disc and experiences complications. As a result of those complications, he or she is no longer able to walk. Another person may have a leg amputated because of recurrent infections. The individual's life has changed significantly in a very short period of time which may create a sense of helplessness and lack of control.

Use of Psychotropic Medications

The use of psychotropic medications among individuals with intellectual disabilities can result in situations that can also be traumatic. Although these medications can be very beneficial, imagine the experience of a non-verbal person with an intellectual disability feeling the effects of a medication. The person feels different. He or she knows something is different but is unable to understand what is happening. Imagine if that individual begins to experience adverse side effects of the medication or the medication results in too much sedation initially. These experiences and physical sensations can be frightening, particularly if the individual is non-verbal and not able to directly communicate his or her internal experiences. Perhaps the person has not been included in the treatment decisions because he or she lacks the verbal skills or the cognitive understanding to consent, or both, or lacks insight into the mental illness. In addition to experiencing potential serious side effects of medications, the individual may also experience withdrawal symptoms from some of the medications if they are discontinued too quickly. These experiences can lead someone to become fearful and confused. I am reminded of an individual who moved out of an institution and into a community residence. The transition was difficult for him, and he began to exhibit some past dangerous behaviors that he had not been exhibiting at the institution for some time. He started threatening to hurt himself, run into traffic, and hurt others. As a result, he was psychiatrically hospitalized, and a new psychotropic medication regimen was introduced. Unfortunately, he had a significant adverse side effect to one of the medications which rendered him almost incapacitated. When I saw him later, he had lost most of his ability to speak, had become incontinent, and had difficulty feeding himself. The experience was not only traumatic for him, but also for the individuals who had been supporting him. Thankfully, he recovered, but to this day he remembers that event and will often say, "I almost died out in the community." Eventually, he returned to the institution and any further discussions about a potential move to a community residence resulted in him becoming highly anxious and resistant.

Chapter 2

Impact of Trauma on the Brain

Before discussing the specifics of trauma-informed care among individuals with intellectual disabilities, it is important to have a basic understanding of the neurobiology of trauma. An understanding of how trauma is created is important in devising strategies for treatment and in understanding the full scope of the impact of trauma. Some challenging behaviors can then be seen not just as "bad behaviors" but as indicators of a nervous system that may be out of balance and dysregulated.

Trauma biology is an advancing area of research which holds much promise in terms of explaining the impact trauma can have on the brain and its implications for healing. Neuroimaging studies such as PET scans (Positron Emission Tomography) and MRIs (Magnetic Resonance Imaging) have been helpful in identifying the parts of the brain which have been structurally and functionally impacted by trauma. Although a comprehensive explanation of the neurobiology of trauma is beyond the scope of this publication, a brief review of the biological alterations it can produce is very important in understanding the impact trauma can have on an individual. A basic understanding of the neurobiology also helps to guide the type of interventions which can be introduced in order to promote healing. It is also important to discuss the changes which can happen in the brain's response to trauma, as it also highlights that people suffering from PTSD are not suffering due to a weakness in character but out of an actual disorder which is occurring at a molecular level.

Based on what has been discovered in the field of neurobiology, understanding the brain structures and its functions can provide an explanation of how trauma is created. An understanding of the neurobiology also provides an explanation for what maintains post-traumatic symptoms. Trauma changes the functioning of the nervous system. However, before exploring how it is changed, it is important to understand the role that the autonomic nervous system plays in trauma. The autonomic nervous system is involved in an individual's responses to her/his environment. It activates part of the nervous system that is often referred to as the "fight or flight" response, and it works without a person's conscious effort. It is continuously active not just when it is in a "fight or flight "mode. In PTSD, the autonomic nervous system fails to discharge the energy from the traumatic experience. Consequently, the system remains out of balance.

The autonomic nervous system is responsible for regulating the function of our internal organs such as the stomach, intestines, and the heart. It also is responsible for controlling some of the muscles. It regulates some of the automatic processes of the body. The autonomic nervous system is composed of the sympathetic nervous and parasympathetic nervous system. The sympathetic nervous system can accelerate the heart rate, raise blood pressure, increase muscle tension, and inhibit the production of insulin in order to maximize a body's fuel sources. The parasympathetic system decreases the heart rate and blood pressure as well as body temperature. It can also increase insulin activity and promote digestion. In essence, the sympathetic nervous (SNS) is the part of the nervous system that "sympathizes" with the situation when it is activated. It is responsible for the "fight or flight" mechanisms. In contrast, the parasympathetic nervous system serves to calm down the body. It is the "cooling" system. It helps us to calm down or cool down and regain our balance. It reverses the effects of the sympathetic nervous system.

When the sympathetic nervous system is dominant there are a number of things that can happen both cognitively and behaviorally. The individual is more likely to be impulsive, irrational, and have difficulty being self-reflective. The individual is not necessarily evaluating behavior from a "good" or "bad" perspective; instead, he or she is reacting. From a neurobiological perspective, most of the behavior which we classify as being impulsive can occur when the body is in this dysregulated state. When the sympathetic nervous system is aroused or is dominant, the nature of someone's thinking process is more immediate and impulsive. In addition, when the brain is sympathetic nervous system dominant, stress hormones are also being released. The brain is actually being bathed in a type of "hormonal and neurochemical cocktail" (Cozolini, 2010). When the brain is being bathed in this cocktail, the individual may have difficulty evaluating his or her actions and regulating emotional responses. This can lead to problematic behaviors such as aggression, anger outbursts, anxiety, hyperactivity, or agitation, if the person is in more of a "fight" mode. When the person is not in a "flight" mode but in a "freeze" mode, more passive behaviors can occur such as emotional distancing, becoming withdrawn, dissociating, etc.

When the autonomic nervous system is dysregulated, the individual is going to respond with survival strategies which are out of proportion to the situation. From a neurobiological perspective, trauma is the body's response to the activation and dysregulation of the body's sympathetic nervous system that has occurred repeatedly or has been in a prolonged state of activation which has then resulted in changes in the person's nervous system (Howard & Crandall, 2007). Therefore, if someone suffers from PTSD, his or her personal history is also asserting itself in dysregulating the system again, and the person is not living in the moment. A memory, a trigger, a flashback, can all bring about these reactions.

The dysregulation that can occur in the nervous system in response to stress and trauma involves a complex interplay of several structures in the brain. As the autonomic nervous system continues to function, there are other parts of the brain which are also involved in the process. For simplicity's sake, we can divide the brain into three sections. The first section is the called the "R complex" which stands for "reptilian" because it is similar to the brains of reptiles and is shared by both reptiles and mammals. It is primitive and instinctive, and it includes the brainstem and cerebellum which helps control the body's basic functions such as temperature, balance, breathing, and heart rate. It is a more primitive part of the brain. It is the oldest in terms of our evolution, and is about survival (Marich, 2014).

The second part of the brain is called the limbic system. The limbic system is often referred to as the "emotional brain." The limbic system structures regulate emotion including a variety of our emotions such as pain, anger, fear, sadness, etc. Additionally, there are two parts of this "emotional brain" that are implicated in PTSD; they are the hippocampus and the amygdala. The autonomic nervous system sends information to the hippocampus, and a major function of the hippocampus has to do with memory. This part of the brain is involved in the forming and organization of memories and our ability to retrieve them. It is responsible for several different types of memory including long-term, short-term, spatial, as well as the forming of new memories. Short-term memories are converted to long-term memories, and trauma can interfere with this process as well as alter it. Traumatic memories may not be fully processed. This may lead to them being too easily activated, producing an over-reactive response by the individual. Since the hippocampus helps the person to discriminate between long term and short term memories, abnormalities in the hippocampus may interfere with this process. For example, if a staff member in a group home says something in a certain tone of voice, it may activate a flashback in one of the residents who had a previous trauma history of emotional abuse. This can lead to an over-reaction and a misinterpretation of the current situation and an overestimation of threat by the individual. The person is reacting to the current situation as if it were the situation occurring in the past and not adequately discriminating past memories from the present.

The autonomic nervous system sends information to the hypothalamus which is another part of the part responsible for regulation or maintaining the status quo. The hypothalamus obtains information from the body and then sends signals back to the autonomic nervous system. It reads body temperature, blood pressure, blood sugar levels, as well as gathering information from the outside world through the individual's five senses. It integrates all of this information and then sends signals back to the body and these signals also go back to the autonomic nervous system. Information also goes to the endocrine system as well to include the pituitary gland which produces hormones. One hormone is particularly important in discussing stress and that is the "stress hormone" known as cortisol. Under stress, the body produces more cortisol which helps to regulate blood pressure and cardiovascular function.

The amygdala, adjacent to the hippocampus, is another area of the brain that can be impacted by severe emotional trauma, and symptoms of PTSD are related to hyperactivity in this area. It is responsible for our emotions and for actions that are motivated by our survival needs. This part of the brain is responsible for the "fight or flight" mode that people have in response to stress and fear. It also activates stress hormones, and it helps to determine if danger is imminent by connecting with the hippocampus which is the database for memories of past experiences of events. As with the hippocampus, there are some studies which have shown a reduced volume in this area in individuals suffering from PTSD as compared to non-PTSD groups (Morey, Gold, & McCarthy, 2012).

The third part of the brain that is involved in this highly complex traffic pattern is the pre-frontal cortex. This area is located in the front of the brain in the outer most layers. This is the area that is responsible for executive functioning. In essence, it functions as the CEO (the chief executive officer) of the brain. It is involved in decision making, problem-solving, self-reflection, moderating behavior, etc., and this part of the brain is also involved in several aspects of memory. The left part of the frontal lobe is involved in the strong memories of events while the right frontal area is able to extract a theme from the events. When an individual is traumatized, basic and more primitive processes become involved and the individual's strong emotional reactions and instincts can override the frontal part of the brain. Lower brain processes are set in motion, and they can override the strength of the cortex which would normally be able to serve an inhibitory function preventing inappropriate behaviors from occurring.

By reviewing these numerous systems, it is apparent that there is a very complex feedback loop in the body and in the brain that responds to danger or threats of danger. Damage to one of these areas can impact other areas. The results of neuroimaging studies on people undergoing stress have shown structural changes can occur in response to trauma either in response to singular traumatic events or continuous threats. As noted by McCarthy (2001), emotional trauma can be a serious threat to an individual's well-being and ability to cope. This can overwhelm the individual's coping mechanisms and compromise their emotional, physical, and cognitive states. The stress response that involves fight, flight, or freeze becomes active rather than returning to its balanced state after the threat has been terminated. This dysregulated, unbalanced state in the nervous system can remain in overdrive and become a more permanent state rather than a temporary one. If this remains in overdrive, it becomes more difficult for the body to sustain it, as it results in high levels of cortisol (a stress hormone) being released which also can inhibit the production of several neurotransmitters (which are known as the chemical messengers in the brain). The release of cortisol from hyperarousal can inhibit the work of several neurotransmitters such as serotonin, norepinephrine, and dopamine. If there are imbalances in these chemicals, it can cause a variety of problems from physical to psychological issues such as impaired memory, poor decision making, pain, obesity, hormonal imbalances, and mood and behavioral disturbances. Antidepressants medications can help to recycle some of the neurotransmitters particularly those impacting serotonin levels. This is why one class of antidepressants, which is referred to as SSRIs (Selective Serotonin Reuptake Inhibitors), is used in the treatment of PTSD.

Although much of the early research in neuropsychology and PTSD focused on deficits in learning and memory, there has been more research which has examined the impact of PTSD on executive functioning skills (Aupperle, Melrose, Stein, & Paulus, 2012). If an individual has difficulty regulating his or her emotions, then it will compromise the individual's executive functioning abilities, and those abilities will not be functioning at full capacity. If emotions can be regulated, then executive functioning abilities improve.

Emotional Regulation and Emotional Dysregulation

If we take into consideration the research from neuroscience regarding the changes in the brain that can occur with trauma, then interventions to promote healing should include strategies to help the nervous system reset itself and return to a balanced state. Consequently, techniques that are aimed at helping individuals regulate their emotions should be part of the treatment plan. Since heightened arousal and persistent negative emotional states are some of the symptoms characterizing posttraumatic stress disorder, they can derail the development of emotional regulation skills. Trauma can interfere with an individual's ability to manage emotions effectively, and strong emotions which are unchecked can have the ability to override executive functioning skills.

Emotional regulation is a term used to refer to a person's ability to manage and control emotional experiences. Emotional regulation strategies can be healthy or unhealthy. For example, listening to music or taking a walk when upset is a healthy coping strategy. Emotional dysregulation refers to an inability to moderate or control emotions in a healthy manner. Examples of unhealthy ways to try and manage emotions or self-soothe could include incidents of overeating or drinking too much. According to Rueda and Pax-Alonso (2013), when emotions are well managed and not dysregulated, executive functioning abilities can be more easily mobilized. The brain is then better able to move from activating its emotional center, which is deep in the brain, to activating aspects of the frontal lobe.

The topic of emotional regulation and dysregulation becomes particularly relevant when supporting individuals with intellectual disabilities with trauma histories because of the studies that suggest that deficits in emotional regulation are already present in this population. If the neurobiological effects of trauma are now added to the equation, in theory, it may be more difficult to heal from trauma. According to Brown, Brown, and Dibiasio (2013), "Approximately one third of adults with intellectual and developmental disabilities have emotion dysregulation and challenging behaviors." Various other researchers have also reported that emotional regulation skill deficits are a contributing factor to behavioral difficulties even though individuals with developmental disabilities and behavioral issues comprise a heterogeneous group (Tyrer et al., 2006; Whitman, 1990). According to a study by Brown et al., (2013), emotional dysregulation was a key variable in challenging behaviors. Consequently, these researchers felt that it was important to focus on improving emotional regulation skills.

Samson et al. (2013) also studied the relationship between emotional dysregulation and developmental disabilities, but the developmental disability that was explored was specifically autism. The study focused on exploring the relationship between emotional regulation skills and the core features of autism which included social and communication deficits, sensory sensitivities, and repetitive and restricted behaviors. According to their findings, children and adolescents with autism spectrum disorder experienced greater difficulties with emotional regulation compared to a typically developing control group. The severity of their symptoms was greater on all of the scales of an 18-item Emotion Dysregulation Index. They found that emotional dysregulation was related to all core features of autism, but it had its greatest association with repetitive behaviors. The interesting aspect of this study was their finding that of all the core features of autism, the core feature which remained the best predictor of emotional dysregulation was repetitive behaviors. According to Samson et al. (2013), "This finding might indicate that individuals with ASD with severe repetitive and restricted symptoms are less able to regulate their emotions due to difficulties inhibiting ongoing behaviors." This finding is consistent with another study conducted by Mazefsky, Pelphrey, and Dahl (2012). While these findings may have important clinical significance, more systematic research is needed in this area. It is interesting to note that Samson, Huber, and Gross (2012) also proposed that "impaired emotional regulation may be a more parsimonious explanation than psychiatric comorbidity for severe behavioral disturbances in Autism Spectrum Disorder."

Given some of the studies that suggest individuals with intellectual disabilities may experience difficulties regulating emotions as a result of the developmental disability itself, consider the additional deficits in emotional regulation that can occur with trauma. In addition to this potentially additive equation, there is evidence from developmental cognitive neuroscience which indicates our ability to regulate emotions are strongly supported by several executive functions, with some studies even suggesting that executive functions can be compromised by a developmental disability (Tottenham, Hare, & Casey, 2011). According to Skoff (2004), there have been a number of studies which have suggested that executive functioning deficits can be found in a number of developmental disorders. These developmental disorders have included not only intellectual disabilities, but also autism spectrum disorder, and other developmental disorders that have genetic causes such as Fragile X (Skoff, 2004).

Executive Functioning Skills and Deficits

Why are executive functioning deficits found among individuals with developmental disabilities? According to Skoff (2004), there are several possible explanations. First, there is a level of structural inter-connectedness between the prefrontal cortex and the rest of the brain. Because of this inter-connectivity, if the brain sustains some type of insult or injury it is likely to impact the functioning in the prefrontal cortex. According to Skoff, "The pre-frontal cortex is the most interconnected part of the brain, with neurons coming from and going to, most other areas in the brain." The disruption or insult to the brain can be at a structural level or a neurochemical level. Skoff also notes, "...there does not have to be specific damage or malfunctioning of the prefrontal cortex for executive deficits to occur: such deficits are possible whenever any part of the brain that functionally interacts with the prefrontal cortex is damaged of disrupted."

If we consider the studies which suggest that individuals with intellectual disabilities have greater difficulties regulating emotions, and we add executive functioning deficits to the equation, imagine the additional impact that trauma to this scenario. Combine all of these factors with various social-environmental conditions that may not be trauma sensitive and may even inadvertently re-traumatize individuals. It becomes no wonder why some individuals with intellectual disabilities develop severe behavioral reputations and are more likely to suffer from psychiatric disorders. We have the sequelae of trauma, combined with the deficits that may accompany the intellectual disability, compounded by environments that may not be trauma sensitive. Such findings would suggest that individuals with intellectual disabilities and a trauma history should have interventions developed which focus on improving emotional regulation skills as primary components of treatment. Although research addressing emotional dysregulation in the general population is expanding, there is less research on emotional regulation training for individuals with intellectual disabilities (McClure, Halpern, Wolper, & Donahue, 2009).

Emotional Regulation Skills Training

Developing these skills may be critical to decreasing some of the behavioral challenges and improving the quality of the lives and relationships for people with intellectual disabilities. There are a variety of methods that can be used to assist individuals in regulating their emotions. Interventions could include incorporating self-soothing strategies such as relaxation training (e.g., diaphragmatic breathing and progressive muscle relaxation exercises), anger management techniques, and problem-solving strategies, as well as some of the specific therapies referenced in later chapters of this book. These strategies would be most appropriate for individuals who are functioning within the mild to moderate range of intellectual functioning. It is important for the body to calm down so that the nervous system does not remain in a heightened level of alert and arousal. However, some of these approaches and strategies which involve more cognitive components may not be appropriate for individuals with intellectual disabilities in the severe and profound ranges. For those individuals, it would be more appropriate to incorporate more self-soothing activities which they find relaxing and calming as well as incorporating more sensory strategies to decrease arousal. Also, there may need to be a greater focus on introducing environmental changes in order to remove any threatening triggers and create a sense of safety and security for them by creating calm environments. This would involve more environmental manipulations. These approaches become more staff (or care provider) intensive requiring staff or care provider training and milieu management.

Developmental Trauma

There is research to suggest that if the trauma occurred early in life, such as in infancy or early childhood, the individual may experience even greater difficulties controlling emotions. If the trauma occurred in infancy or early childhood, this can further shake the very foundation of the individual's ability to self-soothe. Studies have shown that if a parent or care provider is unresponsive or unavailable to an infant during early development, it can contribute to difficulties in the child's ability to self-soothe. These deficits can then be carried over into adulthood. According to Sroufe (1979), when an infant is upset and cries, a caretaker usually comes to provide care and soothe the infant's distress. This allows an opportunity for the baby's nervous system, which is aroused during the periods of distress, to calm down. Gradually, through the consistent presence of a care taker providing relief and soothing a child's emotions, the child is better able to tolerate more intensive emotions which do not lead to periods of emotional disorganization and internal chaos. This research is particularly relevant to individuals with intellectual disabilities due to some of the statistics that have indicated that approximately 25% of children who have disabilities have acquired those due to abuse with 52% of neglected children acquiring a permanent disability (Baladerian, 2013). Let us consider, for example, an individual with a mild intellectual disability who was removed from his parents' care in early childhood due to significant abuse and neglect. He is placed in a series of foster homes, and due to his escalating behavioral challenges he is eventually admitted to an adolescent residential treatment facility. While there, he is surrounded by highly assaultive peers, and he becomes a victim of assault. Is it any wonder that the individual is now known for his impulsive acts of self-harm and aggression towards others? He is easily agitated by events and has difficulty calming down when he is upset. Emotional dysregulation has become a major contributor to his impulsive behaviors. If these behaviors are considered outside of the additional influence of trauma, it runs the risk of misunderstanding his motivations and needs. It is not surprising then to find that this young man has had a history of numerous admissions to psychiatric hospitals. His trauma profile, combined with these other variables, has led to greater and greater interpersonal difficulties for him and a poorer quality of life. His difficulties in self-regulation and its accompanying behaviors may be the result of excessive and prolonged activation of his autonomic nervous system. The accumulation of traumas did not give his body the opportunity to re-establish a balance and to heal. His difficulties controlling his emotions (i.e., his emotional dysregulation) have become a contributor to his impulsive behaviors, and those behaviors may occur at the slightest of provocations.

It is important to assess for any developmental traumas an individual with an intellectual disability may have experienced and to consider the individual's developmental history. Such information may help to explain some of the behaviors from a physiological perspective. Understanding patterns and history is important in trying to identify a trauma profile and this identification can help to ensure that appropriate and effective treatment is provided.

Chapter 3

Diagnosis of PTSD and Trauma-Based Reactions in Individuals with Developmental Disabilities

In order to fully understand the construct of posttraumatic stress disorder, it is helpful to take a quick glance at its evolutionary timeline. This journey includes a basic review of the introduction to the reference guide used by mental health professionals for diagnosing psychiatric disorders, *The Diagnostic and Statistical Manual of Mental Disorders -DSM-5* (American Psychiatric Association, 2013) and its evolution throughout the past 65 years.

HISTORICAL REFERENCES TO PTSD

While the term "posttraumatic stress disorder" did not come into existence until 1980, some of its symptoms have been described for centuries. The Greek historian, Herodotus, described symptoms of emotional strain seen in a soldier battling one of the Persian invasions. During the American Civil War, a physician named Jacob Mendes Da Costa studied the reactions of hundreds of soldiers. He described a variety of symptoms among the soldiers including physical complaints as well as exhaustion which he attributed to the physical demands of combat. The symptoms became known as Da Costa's syndrome. This was replaced by the term "a soldier's heart" in the 20th century. Among the 20th century battlefields beginning in World War I, the term "shell shock" was used to describe a constellation of symptoms including sleep disturbances and anxiety, as well as several other symptoms experienced by some soldiers who had seen combat. These reactions were believed to have been caused by the explosion of artillery shells which were thought to cause lesions in the brain. However, as more solders who had not been around artillery fire reported the same symptoms, the thinking began to change and the term "shell shock" was changed to "war neurosis." During World War II, these symptoms were replaced by the term "combat stress reaction" (CSR) which was also referred to as "battle fatigue" or "combat exhaustion." Battle fatigue accounted for many of the military discharges during World War II. It was beginning to be viewed as a legitimate disorder with treatment consisting of rest, sedation, and even in some cases the use of hypnosis. This was followed by a very high percentage of psychiatric casualties during the Korean War (250 per 1000 per year)

(Ritchie, 2002) and followed by prevalence rates of PTSD ranging between 15.6% and 17.1% among those who served in the Persian Gulf War and the Iraq War (Hoge et al., 2004). Treatment began to focus on returning the individuals to combat quickly by allowing them to rest and having them return to their battle stations with a minimum of delay.

Outside of the battlefield, the origins of some of the diagnostic criteria for PTSD could also be found in the early writings of Sigmund Freud. As noted by Wilson (1994), "Freud's original model of neurosis, known as Seduction Theory, was a post-traumatic paradigm which placed emphasis on external stressor events...Freud's thinking influenced both the DSM-I and II classification of stress response syndromes as transient reactive processes." Freud's seduction theory which he presented in the mid-1890's posited that the origins of hysteria were the result of early childhood sexual abuse. Repressed memories about the events were responsible for hysteria and the symptoms of "obsessional neurosis." He later abandoned this theory and concluded that the memories were not based in reality but were the result of imaginary fantasies (Jahoda, 1977).

THE DIAGNOSTIC AND STATISTICAL MANUAL OF MENTAL DISORDERS

DSM-I

The idea of a combat stress reaction was more formally identified and addressed among mental health practitioners when it was initially introduced in the DSM-I in 1952. The DSM-I was the first manual of mental disorders used to diagnose psychiatric conditions (American Psychiatric Association, 1952). The diagnostic equivalent of PTSD in this manual was referred to as "Gross Stress Reaction." Many Vietnam War veterans were given this diagnosis, and it was considered to be of a short duration.

DSM-II

In the next version of the manual, the DSM-II, which was published in 1968 by the American Psychiatric Association, the equivalent of posttraumatic stress disorder was known as an "Adjustment Reaction of Adult Life." The DSM-II listed three examples of an "adjustment reaction" including a prisoner facing execution, an unwanted pregnancy accompanied by depression and hostility, and fear associated with military combat. It was a very simplistic diagnosis without a description of clinical features that now comprise the most current diagnosis of PTSD.

DSM-III

In 1980, posttraumatic stress disorder (PTSD) was introduced in the DSM-III as a formal diagnosis. The writers of the DSM-III (American Psychiatric Association, 1980) expanded its definition to include the experiences of survivors of other traumas such as abuse, rape, natural disasters, and not just combat experiences. In the DSM-III formulation, a traumatic event was defined as a catastrophic event or stressor that was outside the range of normal human experiences. The developers of the original diagnosis of PTSD considered the traumatic events to be very different from other stressful events which may occur more commonly in life such as illness, financial diffi-

culties, separation, or divorce. If a reaction to more common stressors caused a functional impairment, it could be categorized as an adjustment disorder and not PTSD. If someone was encountering a stressful event, but it was not out of the ordinary, the thinking in the field was that it was not likely to exceed the individual's capacity to cope because it was not a "traumatic stressor." There was an emphasis placed on the type of stressful event the individual encountered. In fact, the diagnosis of PTSD could not be made without one criterion being the "stressor criterion." The individual needed to be exposed to an event that would be considered traumatic. Additional diagnostic criteria included a re-experiencing of the trauma by either recurrent or intrusive recollections, reoccurring dreams of the event, or a sudden feeling or acting as if the event were occurring. There were also criteria that included a numbing of responsiveness or a reduced involvement with the external world evidenced by either a diminished interest in activities, constricted affect, or a feeling of detachment from others. In addition, two of the following six symptoms needed to be present after the trauma occurred that were not present before:
1. Hyper alertness or an exaggerated startle response
2. Sleep disturbances
3. Survivor guilt
4. Difficulties with memory or concentration
5. Avoidance of activities that brought back memories of the trauma
6. Intensification of symptoms when exposed to events that were similar to the traumatic event

In the DSM-III, the diagnosis of PTSD was divided into two types which included an acute form and a chronic or delayed form. In the acute form, the onset of symptoms was within six months of the trauma with a duration of less than six months. In the chronic or delayed form, symptoms lasted longer than six months, and the onset was delayed and occurred at least six months after the trauma.

DSM-III-R

The diagnostic criteria for PTSD outlined in the DSM-III was revised when the DSM-III-R was introduced in 1987 by the American Psychiatric Association. According to the DSM-III-R, "The essential feature of the diagnosis of PTSD was the development of characteristic symptoms following a psychologically distressing event that is outside the range of usual human experience (i.e., outside the range of such common experiences as simple bereavement, chronic illness, business losses, and marital conflict). The stressor producing this syndrome would be markedly distressing to almost anyone and is usually experienced with intensive fear, terror, and helplessness." In addition to the "stressor criterion," the traumatic experience needed to be "persistently re-experienced" either through distressing dreams, intrusive thoughts, flashbacks, etc. The individual also needed to experience a "persistent avoidance of stimuli associated with the trauma or numbing of general responsiveness" as well as at least two of six symptoms of increased arousal. In total, there were 17 diagnostic symptoms identified, and the individual needed to experience six symptoms from three major clusters that included increased physiological arousal that was not present before the trauma, forms of re-experiencing the event, and avoidance reactions or a numbness associated with the traumatic event. These symptoms must have occurred for a minimum of at least one month. There was a qualifier that stated it may be a case of PTSD of delayed onset if the symptoms did not appear until at least six months after being experiencing.

It is interesting to note that it was not until the DSM–III-R (American Psychiatric Association, 1987) was published that the mental health field recognized that PTSD could develop in children as well as adults. Initially, diagnostic criteria for children were simply a downward extension from observations made in adults. When the fourth version of the *Diagnostic and Statistical Manual,* the DSM-IV-TR- (American Psychiatric Association, 2000) was introduced, it included specific descriptions of how symptoms may manifest in children. At that time it was noted that a child's response to a traumatic event may be manifested as disorganized or agitated behavior, rather than intense fear or horror. Children may also manifest traumatic reactions through repetitive play and through frightening dreams.

DSM-IV

In 1994, the DSM-IV was published by the American Psychiatric Association and it changed the criteria for a diagnosis of PTSD. The changes represented a refinement over the diagnostic criteria that were outlined in previous versions of the Statistical and Diagnostic manuals. In earlier versions of the manual, the traumatic stressor was defined as a source of stress outside the range of usual experiences that anyone would find significantly distressing. This technically could eliminate stressful and traumatic experiences which may occur more commonly, such as domestic abuse or child abuse. The DSM-IV expanded the definition of traumatic stress to include indirect threats to one's life or well-being, as well as direct threats to the individual, producing a sense of severe helplessness, horror, or fear. To meet the "exposure to the trauma" criterion, an individual must have either experienced or witnessed events that involved the threat of death, or serious damage to an individual's physical integrity or to the physical integrity of others. The person's response must have included intense fear, helplessness, or horror. Consequently, the traumatic event could have been experienced by the individual directly, or the individual could have witnessed it occurring to someone else and as a result felt horrified, helpless, and fearful. This was followed by three symptom clusters that included some type of intrusive recollections, avoidant/numbing symptoms, and hyper-arousal symptoms. In addition, the event needed to be re-experienced in one or more ways such as through distressing dreams, physiological reactivity, or distressing thoughts. A persistent avoidance of stimuli associated with the trauma and numbing of general responsiveness was also needed for the diagnosis. In addition, symptoms of increased arousal needed to present. The duration of symptoms was also specified (i.e., acute, chronic, or delayed onset). These symptoms must have caused significant distress or impairment in the individual's life.

DSM-IV-TR

In 2000, the DSM-IV-TR was introduced by the American Psychiatric Association and referred to as the "text revision" of the DSM-IV. In this revision, the vast majority of diagnostic categories remained the same. One of the biggest changes was the fact that diagnoses were accompanied by a five part axial system. It provided a multiaxial diagnosis with the following content identified on each axis: Axis I: Psychiatric disorders; Axis II: Personality disorders and developmental disabilities; Axis III: Medical and physical conditions; Axis IV: Major or environmental stressors that may be affecting the individual; and Axis V: The Global Assessment of Functioning (GAF). The GAF was a scale that provided a subjective, numerical rating used by mental health professionals to estimate an individual's level of social, occupational, and psychological functioning.

DSM-5

In 2013, the diagnostic criteria for PTSD underwent yet another revision by the APA with the publication of the DSM-5. In this new manual, a number of changes were made to the PTSD diagnostic criteria which consisted of evidence-based revisions (i.e., based on research findings). One of the biggest changes occurred in the category of disorders in which posttraumatic stress disorder had been included. Prior to the DSM-5, posttraumatic stress disorder was categorized as a form of an anxiety disorder. However, further examination and research indicated that it is not just a fear-based disorder as indicated in the DSM-III and the DSM-IV. Posttraumatic stress can also present with various mood states such as a dysphoric mood, a lack of interest in activities or withdrawal, and not just anxiety. It can also manifest in behavioral symptoms such as angry outbursts or reckless and self-destructive behaviors. As a result of these research-based changes, PTSD is now classified in the DSM-5 under a new category called *Trauma and Stressor-Related Disorders*.

Since PTSD it is still preceded by exposure to a traumatic or otherwise adverse environmental event in the DSM-5, it is still a unique disorder as compared to the rest of the disorders because it is the result of a specific environmental event. It requires that a specific event criterion is met in order to diagnosis this disorder. In the DSM-5, there are three categories of trauma that are listed: an actual incident or threat of physical injury, sexual violation, or death. Exposure to any one of these events must be experienced in one or more of the following ways in order to meet the first criterion for the diagnosis:

1. Either through directly experiencing the event
2. By witnessing any one of these events as it is happening to someone else
3. Learning that the traumatic event has occurred to either a "close family member or close friend" – This also specifies that in cases of actual or threatened death of a family member or friend, the event(s) must have been violent or accidental.
4. Experiencing repeated or extreme exposure to aspects of the traumatic event(s)

It specifically excludes exposure to these events if it occurred through television, electronic media, or pictures, unless the exposure occurred as part of one's job. One of the difficulties with this criterion is that it is very limiting. The indirect exposure qualifier states that the person who was traumatized indirectly by learning about an event that happened to someone else had to be either a close friend or a close family member. Another difference in Criterion A, as compared to DSM-IV-TR, is the removal of the requirement that the person must have experienced emotional reactions to the traumatic event that included fear, helplessness, or horror.

The core symptoms in the DSM-5 were also expanded and now include four categories rather than three. A symptom of persistent negative alterations in mood and cognition was added to the three core categories of symptoms which included the re-experiencing the event, avoidance behaviors, and arousal symptoms. Additional criteria are required before a diagnosis of PTSD can be given. These include the following: the symptoms must have been present for one month or longer; the symptoms must cause significant impairment or distress; and the symptoms must not be due to a substance such as alcohol or to a medical condition.

The DSM-5 also lists separate criteria for the diagnosis of posttraumatic stress disorder in children who are 6-years-old or younger.

In the DSM-5, under this new category of *Trauma and Stress Related Disorders*, PTSD is listed as a diagnosis along with the following five other possible diagnoses:

- *Acute stress disorder* – The main difference between acute stress disorder and PTSD is the duration of the symptoms. Symptoms of acute stress disorder resolve within several days to four weeks after the event. If the symptoms continue beyond the four weeks and impair functioning, the diagnosis may change to PTSD. The diagnosis of acute stress disorder also differs from PTSD in that it requires 9 out of 14 symptoms from 5 categories that include dissociation, negative mood, intrusion, arousal, and avoidance. This diagnostic category is associated more with a specific trauma rather than a chronic exposure to traumatic stress.
- *Reactive attachment disorder*
- *Disinhibited social engagement disorder*
- *Adjustment disorders*
- *Trauma or stressor related-disorders not elsewhere classified*

THE DM-ID-DIAGNOSTIC MANUAL-INTELLECTUAL DISABILITY AND THE DM-ID-2

In 2007, the National Association for the Dually Diagnosed in association with the American Psychiatric Association published a diagnostic manual that was a modification of the DSM-IV-TR specifically designed for individuals with intellectual disabilities (Fletcher, Loschen, Stavrakaki, & First, 2007). It was referred to as the DM-ID – *Diagnostic Manual – Intellectual Disability (DM-ID): A Clinical Guide for Diagnosis of Mental Disorders in Persons with Intellectual Disability*. It was the first diagnostic manual that offered adaptations of psychiatric diagnoses in the *Diagnostic and Statistical Manual*, the DSM-IV-TR, for people with intellectual disabilities. This was written in response to the complications and challenges that can arise in applying the same diagnostic criteria that are used to diagnose psychiatric disorders in the general population to individuals with intellectual disabilities. Given the communication deficits, physical limitations, cognitive limitations, and adaptive deficits that can accompany intellectual disabilities, the symptom presentation is sometimes atypical and/or masked. The DM-ID describes some of the differences in symptoms that may be seen at the various levels of intellectual functioning. For example, at the lower ranges of cognitive functioning such as severe and profound intellectual disabilities, the individual who is experiencing posttraumatic stress disorder is more likely to exhibit more overt behaviors in response to re-experiencing aspects of the traumatic event such as self-injurious behaviors or periods of agitation or aggression (Fletcher et al., 2007; Razza & Tomasulo, 2005). There may be more incidents of behavioral acting out in response to the trauma among individuals with lower levels of cognitive functioning. They may also exhibit more bizarre or disorganized behaviors which are sometimes confused or misinterpreted as signs of psychosis when they may be re-enactments of the trauma (Razza & Tomasulo, 2005). Since the individual may lack the verbal skills at the lower levels of intellectual functioning, it hinders the person's ability to verbalize symptoms such as experience with flashbacks or intrusive memories. Thus, the behaviors among individuals with severe to profound ID can look more confusing or bizarre to others because they are not being viewed as responses to intrusive memories or re-experiences of aspects of the trauma. In addition, the DM-ID discusses how the range of traumatic life events may be more extensive for individuals with intellectual disabilities than included in the event criterion for PTSD listed in the DSM-5.

According to the DM-ID (Fletcher et al., 2007), the equivalent of an avoidance of the stimuli associated with the trauma among individuals with intellectual disabilities may appear somewhat different than in the general population. Among individuals with mild to moderate levels of ID, the person's attempts to avoid situations that re-stimulate memories may be termed "non-compliant" behavior. Among individuals with more severe levels of ID (i.e., severe and profound ranges), their avoidance behaviors may also be viewed as incidents of non-compliance but they may also isolate as expressions of feelings of detachments or estrangements from others. In response to the traumatic event, there may be an increase in agitation among individuals with mild to moderate ID as compared to the general population. Among individuals whose intellectual functioning is in the severe to profound range, agitated behavior may be more commonplace as compared to the general population.

DM-ID-2

Since the DM-ID's original publication in 2007, it has been updated and modified and it is now the DM-ID-2 (Fletcher, Barnhill, & Cooper, 2016) in response to the new diagnostic manual, the DSM-5. With regard to the diagnosis of PTSD among individuals with intellectual disabilities, the following points and adaptations have been noted in the DM-ID-2:

- Individuals with intellectual disabilities continue to show an increased vulnerability to developing PTSD than the general population.
- Among individuals with intellectual disabilities in the mild range, the symptom presentation for PTSD resembles more of the symptoms seen in the general population. Individuals with lower levels of cognitive functioning (i.e., in the severe and profound range) may exhibit a range of behaviors and symptoms that may not be seen the general population. This can make the identification of PTSD more complicated. Among individuals with more severe and profound intellectual disabilities, incidents of behavioral acting out are more common.
- Individuals with intellectual disabilities experience greater exposure to conditions that may contribute to the development of PTSD. According to the DM-ID-2, with regard to the event criterion (Criterion A) for the diagnosis

of PTSD, "Typically the lower the developmental age, the lower the threshold for what qualifies as traumatic." Therefore, the event criterion for the general population may be too limiting for individuals with intellectual disabilities.

SIGNS AND SYMPTOMS OF PTSD IN INDIVIDUALS WITH ID AND DIAGNOSTIC COMPLICATIONS

Diagnosing posttraumatic stress disorder among individuals with intellectual disabilities can be a challenging process. In the general population, if individuals have been exposed to very stressful events, they can report their reactions and symptoms. There are also a variety of standardized tests available for the general population to measure PTSD symptoms and event reporting which can assist in diagnosing PTSD. However, these conditions are often lacking among individuals with intellectual disabilities, and there are a variety of factors that can complicate the diagnostic process among this population. These include the following:

- The individual may lack the expressive language skills to self-report symptoms. At the lower levels of intellectual functioning (i.e., profound and severe) the individual is usually non-verbal. Therefore, some symptoms can only be inferred by observing changes in behavior.
- The level of cognitive functioning may interfere with the individual's ability to accurately report their experiences making it difficult to tell if their symptoms meet the diagnostic criteria for PTSD.
- Often individuals with intellectual disabilities have histories of multiple placements and records are not available that provide documentation of the traumatic events. Consequently, the individual's complete history with regard to the origin and to the evolution of the symptoms may be unknown.
- An individual's behavioral challenges may be misunderstood and the motives for the behavior misattributed. For example, an avoidance of activities is mislabeled as non-compliance when it may be a desire to avoid aspects of the environment that re-stimulate traumatic memories.
- Claims of abuse may be discounted by staff or care providers due to an absence of corroborating data or incomplete records, or as a result of a person's history.
- The symptoms may be mistakenly attributed to the developmental disability rather than being considered symptomatic of an underlying psychiatric disorder.
- There is a lack of standardized measures to assist in diagnosing PTSD.
- The recency of the traumatic event is also a factor that may complicate the presentation. If the individual's behaviors changed soon after experiencing a traumatic or stressful event, it may be easier to consider trauma related reactions or even a diagnosis of PTSD, provided the symptoms are debilitating enough. However, if abuse or another form of trauma occurred years ago, it may be more difficult to discern whether or not the person's behaviors are related to, or influenced by, the traumatic events. In addition, behavioral challenges that may have started in response to trauma may have been reinforced by other factors. This could result in the behavior becoming a multi-deter-

mined one and not a purely trauma-based reaction. For example, an individual with profound intellectual functioning becomes aggressive in response to meeting a male staff who resembled someone who previously abused her. In response to that aggressive act, the staff member left her alone, and she was also able to escape a task she didn't want to do such as change her clothes. The aggressive behavior may now be maintained by several different factors. If she becomes aggressive people will leave her alone, and she may also not have to perform a task or an activity she doesn't want to perform.
- The developmental level of the individual can affect the presentation of symptoms resulting in symptoms which may be masked or atypical.

Among these obstacles to diagnosing PTSD among individuals with intellectual disabilities, the individual's developmental level can make it more difficult to identify an event as traumatic. The developmental level of the individual also affects the presentation of the symptoms. According to Tomasulo and Razza (2007), the developmental level can influence how the "trauma-related sequelae" are exhibited. At the lower levels of intellectual functioning (i.e., the profound and severe level), the symptoms may be different from what is normally seen in the general adult population and may resemble more of the behaviors or reactions usually seen in children suffering from PTSD. For example, in the general population, young children may exhibit regressed behaviors or aggression (Wilgosh, 1993). Among very young children in the general population, symptoms may include the following:
- Fear of being separated from their parent
- Regression in skills such as toileting skills
- Irritability
- Aggression
- Compulsive play with repetitive themes surround the trauma
- Sleep difficulties and nightmares
- Physical complaints with no medical causes
- New fears, phobias, or anxieties

According to Hieger (2012), children differ in how they may exhibit signs and symptoms of PTSD which includes a time distortion. Sometimes children will not recall the events in the proper time sequence. Hamblen & Barnett (2009) also note that children may reenact aspects of the trauma behaviorally.

Researchers (van der Kolk, 1996) have also noted that an individual's developmental level has a significant impact on his or her ability to cope with traumatic experiences. In addition, individuals whose cognitive abilities lie within the lower levels of intellectual functioning are more likely to experience potentially traumatic events and the effects of PTSD (Breslau, Lucia, & Alvarado, 2006) and a greater severity of PTSD symptoms (McNally & Shin, 1995).

With regard to developmental considerations, of special concern is the constellation of symptoms that may occur when the trauma consists of abuse and neglect of infants and children at very young ages. As noted by Levy (1999), one of the most debilitating consequences of disruptive and disordered attachments among children is difficulties the children may experience in regulating and modulating their emotions. This can lead to impulsive behaviors and behaviors that result from deficits in their abilities to regulate their emotions. Such difficulties can lead to challenging behaviors such as aggression towards others and self-injury. Difficulties in modulating emotions and impulses can then lead to a myriad of psychosocial problems. Secure attachments during childhood are critical in order for children to learn self-control.

Imagine early childhood abuse and neglect and its consequences and its sequelae coupled with the challenges inherent in having an intellectual disability. Add to this equation, an accumulation of traumas later in life or multiple adverse life events. This can lead to severe behavioral reputations, psychiatric hospitalizations, multiple placements, numerous psychotropic medications, and multiple psychiatric diagnoses.

Symptoms of posttraumatic stress disorder among older children in the general population may involve more problems with conduct. Manifestations could include self-injurious behavior, difficulties at school, and even substance abuse issues (McCarthy, 2001). According to McCarthy (2001), this emphasizes the importance of viewing the symptoms of PTSD within the context of the individual's developmental level including the emotional and cognitive levels of development.

Among adults who have developmental disabilities and PTSD whose intellectual disabilities were in the higher ranges of cognitive functioning (i.e., mild to moderate), Ryan (1994) noted they tend to report flashbacks, nightmares, hypervigilance, and other signs of increased arousal. They reported distress and active attempts to avoid reminders of the traumatic event. According to Wieland, Warenaar, Dautovic, and Zitman (2013), individuals with intellectual disabilities in the mild range also share some of the same responses that occur in the general adult population including sleep disturbances such as nightmares and agitation. McCarthy (2001) noted that aggression is one of the most common presenting symptoms. However, McCarthy also emphasized the importance of being aware that among individuals with intellectual disabilities there may be a wide range of symptoms or behaviors that are symptomatic of possible PTSD. In addition to the sleep disturbances and agitation, there may also be a depressed mood, incidents of self-harm or self-injurious behavior, defiant behavior, distractibility, emotional outbursts, and aggression.

Tomasulo and Razza (2007) also identified a list of symptoms that include cognitive and behavioral symptoms that may be present in individual with intellectual disabilities who have PTSD. They include the following:

Cognitive symptoms
- Confusion
- Concentration difficulties
- Difficulties with memory including difficulty remembering aspects of the traumatic event
- Difficulties making decisions
- Difficulty talking about the traumatic event

Behavioral symptoms
- Sleep disturbances
- Nightmares
- Fatigue
- Spontaneous crying
- Agitation

- Physical complains such as digestive problems and headaches
- Difficulties facing certain aspects of the trauma that can be manifested in avoidance behaviors

Other researchers have also proposed various behavioral equivalents for PTSD that may be present in individuals with intellectual disabilities, particularly at the lower levels of cognitive functioning. However, there is still a lack of empirical evidence for some of the behavioral equivalents for PTSD among this population, and some of the descriptions are based on clinical observations and anecdotal information. According to Tomasulo and Razza (2007), there is still some evidence that at the lower levels of cognitive functioning PTSD may be manifested by an increased likelihood of exhibiting agitated or disorganized behavior.

In supporting individuals with intellectual disabilities throughout the years, this author has also observed some of the following behaviors in individuals who have significant trauma histories consisting of physical and/or sexual abuse:

- Verbalizing statements that people can't be trusted
- Hiding in closets or enclosed spaces in response to certain noises
- Episodes of rage or intense irritability
- A pattern of increasing behavioral challenges that occur around specific times of the year which can signal anniversary reactions of loss
- Scanning the environment
- Anger accompanied by statements that people are trying to control them
- Asking to see what someone may be writing about them
- Outbursts or anger if they see someone reading their chart
- What appears to be paranoia about contacting previous care providers or institutions for history
- Exhibiting self-defensive postures such as raising hands above the head in a self-protective stance as someone approaches or placing their hands over their genitalia
- Quick startle response
- Nervousness as people approach or get near
- Aggression directed to individuals that share similar characteristics
- Loss of language in someone who previously could speak
- Aggression towards new people
- Aggression directed towards medical personnel
- Regressions in ability to communicate (e.g., mutism)

This list has been based on clinical experiences and these behaviors have not been empirically studied as possible indicators of PTSD. Of concern in witnessing some of these behaviors have been the reactions sometimes expressed by staff or care providers. It has not been uncommon in this author's experience to have care providers identify some of these behaviors as simply being "attention-seeking" in origin. It is possible that a behavior that was once exhibited for a specific reason, such as a response to trauma, can also occur in response to other motivations. For example, a person may have become aggressive in response to a trauma trigger but then learned their response resulted in people leaving them alone and lowering tasks demands. This could lead to future incidents of aggression as a means to escape a task demand.

However, it is important that care providers also remain sensitive to the fact that challenging behaviors may be occurring in response to trauma-related psychological distress. Clinicians need to adapt to the many ways that trauma-related responses can be exhibited among individuals with intellectual disabilities.

SUBTHRESHOLD PTSD

Given the limitations in the "event criterion" (Criterion A) for PTSD in the DSM-5, the topic of subthreshold PTSD becomes an important one among individuals with intellectual disabilities who have experienced trauma. Subthreshold PTSD refers to the experiencing of symptoms after experiencing a traumatic event(s) but the symptoms fall short of meeting the full criteria for a diagnosis of PTSD. Subthreshold PTSD has also been referred to as subsyndromal PTSD and partial PTSD. According to some researchers (Mylle & Maes, 2004; Pietrzak, Goldstein, Southwick, & Grant, 2011), partial PTSD is commonly defined as having at least one symptom of PTSD from Criteria, B, C, and D, and the symptoms continue to occur at least one month after the traumatic event.

Among the general population, researchers have debated the validity of the concept of subthreshold PTSD since it was first discussed in reference to Vietnam War veterans (Cukor, Wyka, Jayasinghe, & Difede, 2010). The debate has centered around concerns that clinicians may be creating a disorder where there is none, and they may be pathologizing a normal reaction to trauma (Cukor et al., 2010; Breslau, Wilcox, Storr, Lucia, & Anthony, 2004). However, if the concept of subthreshold PTSD is rejected, it runs the risk of neglecting those individuals who may be experiencing some impairments in their day-to-day functioning and who are distressed by their experiences and symptoms (Jakupcak et al., 2007).

A number of studies have been conducted in the general population that have investigated the rates and the associated impairments among individuals whose symptoms do not meet full PTSD criteria. They have compared these findings to individuals whose symptoms meet full criteria and to those individuals reporting no symptoms. Cukor et al. (2010) studied the responses of 3360 workers assigned to Ground Zero after the 9/11 attacks. They investigated the rates of subthreshold PTSD and associated impairments and compared those impairments to individuals who met full criteria for PTSD and to those with no symptoms. Their study was a prospective one which studied individual's responses over the course of three years. At the Time 1 interval, they found that 9.7% of the individuals in their study met the criteria for subthreshold PTSD. Among the three groups of individuals (i.e., the no PTSD group, subthreshold PTSD group, or full PTSD group), there were significantly different levels of impairments. At Time 2, 29% of their initial sample with subthreshold PTSD continued to meet either criterion for subthreshold or full criteria for PTSD, and this was true for 24.5% of their initial sample at the third interval. According to Cukor et al. (2010), the study adds credence to the clinical importance of subthreshold PTSD and that this subclinical form of PTSD may also produce significant and longstanding impairments. It also highlights some of the clinical differences between subthreshold PTSD and PTSD.

Other studies have also been conducted in an attempt to understand whether or not the construct of subthreshold PTSD has utility and clinical significance. Most of the studies that have been conducted have found increased levels of impairment among individuals with subthreshold PTSD as compared to control groups of individuals with no PTSD symptoms. However, it has also been found that the levels of impairment among individuals who met full criteria for PTSD are greater than for those with subthreshold PTSD (Jakupcak et al., 2007; Marshall, Beebe, Oldham, & Zaninelli, 2001). Other studies have also found higher rates of suicidal ideation (Marshall et al., 2001) and alcohol use (Adams, Boscarino, & Galea, 2006) among individuals with subthreshold PTSD than among the general population. Jakupcak et al. (2007) also found subthreshold PTSD to be associated with increased anger and aggression. Rosenberg et al. (2001) found that subthreshold symptoms can exacerbate any existing psychiatric conditions such as anxiety or depression.

Although there is a lack of research studying the impact of subthreshold PTSD among individuals with intellectual disabilities, the construct of subthreshold PTSD may be particularly important for this population due to a variety of reasons. These include the following:

- Individuals with intellectual disabilities are vulnerable to a wide range of events that may be traumatic which may not meet the specific event criterion for a PTSD diagnosis. However, the individual may still be traumatized by the events and experience a myriad of symptoms and psychological distress that can impact behavior.
- Symptoms that meet the full criteria for PTSD may not be easily identifiable among this population due to communication deficits, cognitive limitations, a lack of social opportunities, and physical limitations, etc. However, symptoms may still be present and affecting the individual's behaviors. Without recognizing the possibility that the behaviors may be reflective of subthreshold PTSD, treatments or interventions may be introduced that are ineffective. For example, if an individual's behavior is mislabeled as attention-seeking in nature, resulting in a strictly behavioral approach, the intervention may be ineffective because it did not take into consideration the behavior's origin in trauma. Some clinicians may overlook the genesis of the behavior as based in trauma, since they could not find enough evidence to support a diagnosis of full PTSD.
- Subthreshold symptoms may be mild, atypical, or even masked in this population similar to some of the symptoms of other psychiatric disorders. This requires an even greater sensitivity on the part of the clinician to subsyndromal symptoms.
- Individuals with intellectual disabilities and unrecognized trauma-based behaviors run the risk of developing behavioral reputations that may make it difficult for them to succeed or meet their needs. This may be particularly true for those individuals whose levels of cognitive impairments are in the profound and severe ranges and whose symptoms may be expressed in behavioral equivalents.
- Increased prevalence rates for psychiatric disorders among this population have been quoted by various researchers. Studies in the general population have identified increased risk for other psychiatric disorders because of subthreshold PTSD (i.e., depression and substance abuse). This could feasibly

increase the risk to an even greater extent that an individual with ID may develop another psychiatric disorder. It is unknown at this time if one of the reasons for the increased risk of psychiatric conditions among this population may, in fact, be a result of unidentified trauma-based reactions and dynamics. There are theories as to why this population has higher prevalence rates of psychiatric disorders than the general population, but they are only hypotheses.

- Subthreshold PTSD may be linked to an increased risk of aggression among this population. Among this population, aggressive behavior is often a reason for receiving discharge notices from placements or for admissions to psychiatric hospitals. If trauma-based reactions are contributors to aggression, then providing interventions specifically geared towards addressing the trauma may decrease the incidents. This could lead to a decrease in the utilization rate of psychiatric hospitals and also lessen the risk of injury to care providers and staff, as well as decrease the risk of failed placements.

Given the findings that partial PTSD in the general population may have a chronic course, and it has a potential to produce functional impairments, as well as impact other disorders, it becomes an important construct to explore. If symptoms of subthreshold PTSD are not recognized and treated early, they may run the risk of eventually meeting the criteria for full PTSD. Therefore, early intervention is important. Consequently, clinicians as well as care providers should remain sensitive to the possibilities that challenging behaviors among this population may have their roots in trauma and may be symptomatic of partial PTSD.

Assessing for Co-Morbidity

Assessing for co-morbidity is assessing for the co-occurrence of another psychiatric condition that may accompany PTSD. With posttraumatic stress disorder there is a high co-occurrence of certain psychiatric conditions such as substance abuse (i.e., alcohol and/or drug use), depressive disorders, anxiety disorders (Kessler, Sonnega, Bromet, Huges, & Nelson, 1995), chronic pain, somatization, and eating disorders among the general population (Kessler et al.; 1995, Rosenberg et al., 2001). Research would indicate that co-morbidity is, "the rule and not the exception" (Brady, Killeen, Brewerton, & Lucerini, 2000) with this disorder. According to Brady, Killeen et al. (2000), the results from epidemiological studies have indicated that the majority of people who have been diagnosed with PTSD also meet the criteria for another psychiatric condition with some even having three or more psychiatric diagnoses. As stated in the DSM-5 (American Psychiatric Association, 2013), individuals with PTSD are 80% more likely to also have at least one other psychiatric diagnosis. Therefore, it is important when any psychiatric diagnosis is present to also ascertain whether or not it is related to trauma, and whether or not any posttraumatic symptoms are also present. For example, avoidance reactions due to trauma can progress to the extent that phobias develop. The individual may then develop an irrational fear of certain situations or objects, and this anxiety and withdrawal could even cause paranoia. Consequently, if the phobia is simply viewed as an irrational fear and not appreciated or identified as being related to trauma, treatment may be not be comprehensive or effective.

The presence of a co-occurring psychiatric disorder can complicate treatment. It can make the identification of PTSD, or any disorder, challenging since it may be difficult to discern which psychiatric condition is primary. In addition, there may be some symptom overlap between some of the disorders such as depressive or anxiety disorders and PTSD that may make the diagnostic process more confusing and challenging. Among individuals with intellectual disabilities who have PTSD, diagnosing secondary psychiatric issues can become considerably more challenging at the lower levels of intellectual functioning (i.e., profound and severe levels).

Most of the research on co-morbid psychiatric conditions and PTSD has come from research among the general population. There is a paucity of systematic research in the psychological and psychiatric literature about the prevalence and type of co-occurring psychiatric conditions with PTSD among individuals with intellectual disabilities. However, it is just as important, if not more important, to determine whether or not other conditions exist in addition to PTSD among this population because of the high prevalence rates of mental illness among them. Treatment of any of psychiatric conditions may be rendered ineffective, and proper treatment can be delayed, if the full diagnostic picture is not identified and addressed. Therefore, it requires a careful evaluation including a thorough history and, in particular, obtaining a trauma history among individuals with intellectual disabilities.

PTSD and Somatic Symptoms

When diagnosing posttraumatic stress disorder, there is an emphasis on the psychological symptoms of the disorder. However, posttraumatic stress disorder can have an impact on an individual's physical health. Sometimes the symptoms of PTSD begin with a presentation of common physical complaints such as headaches or digestive problems. The connection between trauma and health conditions was noted in the ACE Study when researchers found strong associations between early childhood trauma and adverse experiences and physical disorders.

There have been numerous studies since the ACE Study which have found that individuals with PTSD are at a greater risk for the development of a number of different physical disorders (Calhoun, Wiley, Dennis, & Beckham, 2009; Friedman, 2000). Boscarino (1997) found that as the severity of the exposure to the trauma increased so did the number of reported health conditions. The health issues were varied and included disorders from several different systems such as digestive, endocrine, musculoskeletal, and circulatory problems. These occurred even after controlling for health behavior. Lauterbach, Rajvee, and Rakow (2005) found that among 5,877 participants in their study who had been diagnosed with PTSD, there was a higher frequency of health problems even after controlling for such variables as gender, co-occurring psychiatric diagnoses, daily stress, health-related behaviors, daily stress, and trauma exposure.

There have been a variety of theories proposed to explain the potential mechanisms for why traumatized individuals experience greater health problems. One explanation is embedded in the diagnosis for PTSD which includes alterations in physiological reactivity and arousal and the imbalances that can occur in the autonomic nervous system. Trauma can also negatively impact the body's hormonal stress response system which can adversely impact health (De Kloet, Karst, & Joels, 2008).

Studies have also shown that chronic stress can compromise immune functioning (McEwen, 2005).

Although there have been numerous studies which have examined the impact that trauma exposure can have on the health of individuals in the general population, there have been a dearth of studies on this topic among individuals with intellectual disabilities. However, if we extrapolate from the findings obtained in these studies to the population of individuals with intellectual disabilities, it is important to be sensitive to their presentation of physical symptoms and health conditions. The self-reporting of physical symptoms, or the presence of various physical conditions, may serve as a cue signaling a trauma history.

There is also the possibility that individuals with intellectual disabilities who are verbal may self-report physical symptoms that cannot be substantiated. This may increase the risk that the person with a trauma history may receive a psychiatric diagnosis from the category of "Somatic Symptoms and Related Disorders." This is a group of disorders in the DSM-5 that are characterized by physical symptoms that are causing an individual significant impairment and distress and may be medically unexplained. The person's reporting of physical symptoms may also be a way of expressing and managing negative emotions and may reflect ongoing distress. For some individuals whose stress symptoms are reflected in physical complaints, they may be unaware of the connection between their somatic symptoms and trauma-related stress. The person may also be resistant to exploring their emotions and maintain their physical symptoms as a way to avoid the emotions. The person may even insist that the physical symptoms require medical attention even in light of medical tests that fail to substantiate their presence. Therefore, it is important to explore the timing of somatic symptoms relative to the events in a person's life.

It is also important to screen for trauma among this population in the midst of increasing physical complaints or physical conditions. This may help to provide clues as to whether or not traumatic stress responses are present. However, before assuming that the reports of physical ailments are expressions of unresolved or unexpressed trauma, it is important to rule out all legitimate medical causes. Ruling out an underlying medical illness is a prerequisite for diagnosing any psychiatric disorder among this population, as well as in the general population. However, this is particularly important when supporting individuals with intellectual disabilities due to some of the language limitations that can occur among this population. In addition, some of the causes of the intellectual disabilities may have their origins in genetic syndromes which may have a constellation of physical disorders as part of the syndrome.

Psychosis and PTSD

The co-occurrence of posttraumatic stress disorder and psychosis is higher than what would be expected for each disorder by itself (Bosson, Reuther, & Cohen, 2011). Among the general population, a substantial percentage of people who suffer from PTSD also experience psychotic symptoms. In the first population-based study to examine the association between PTSD and positive signs of psychosis, Sareen, Cox, Goodwin, and Asmundson (2005) from the Universities of Manitoba, Columbia, and Regina interviewed 5,877 participants from throughout the United States. Positive symptoms of psychosis included hallucinations and delusions, whereas, negative symptoms of psychosis included a blunting of affect, withdrawal, lack of motivation, etc. They found that among their sample 52% of people who reported having PTSD at some time in their life also reported experiencing a positive symptom of psychosis. In their study, they found that 27.5 % of the participants believed people were spying on them, 19.8% believed they were seeing things that other people were not seeing, 12.4% thought they could hear other people's thoughts, and 10.3% were having olfactory hallucinations. The researchers also found the risk of experiencing positive symptoms of psychosis increased as the number of PTSD symptoms increased. The statistics for the prevalence of psychosis among individuals with PTSD have varied per study, but, overall, research has shown a high incidence of co-morbidity between the two disorders (Kilcommons & Morrison, 2005; Strakowski, Keck, McElroy, Lonczak, & West, 1995).

There have been several hypotheses to account for these findings. Coentre and Power (2011) stated that there is evidence to demonstrate that both of the psychiatric disorders may emerge from trauma. Individuals with schizophrenia, which is a form of psychosis, have often been found to have trauma histories (Razza, 1997). Another possibility is that the diagnosis of PTSD increases the risk of psychosis. In addition, researchers have also proposed that PTSD with psychotic features may be a subtype of PTSD and reflect a more severe form of the disorder (Lindley, Carlson, & Sheikh, 2000). Other researchers have suggested that PTSD with psychotic features may be a misdiagnosis when, in fact, the person is really exhibiting prodromal symptoms of schizophrenia (Oconghaile & DeLisi, 2015). Extreme PTSD can look like psychosis. For example, if an individual is having a flashback from a traumatic event, depending upon the strength of the flashback, it can lead to a dissociative episode whereby the individual is no longer responding to the reality of the situation but to a past reality. Consequently, flashbacks, intrusive thoughts, and memories from PTSD must be differentiated from hallucinations, delusions, and other perceptual disturbances that can occur in various forms of psychosis such as schizophrenia. With posttraumatic stress disorder, changes can occur in the thought patterns of individuals in response to traumatic stress making it sometimes difficult to discern aspects of PTSD from psychosis.

Diagnosing psychosis in individuals with intellectual disabilities can be a challenging task with the challenges increasing as the level of intellectual functioning decreases. At the lower levels of cognitive functioning, the individual is usually non-verbal or primarily non-verbal and not able to describe his/her perceptual experiences. The clinician is then left to make inferences based on observations of the individual and information gathered from others familiar with the person.

Ryan (1994) proposed the following list of behaviors which may be seen in individuals with intellectual disabilities who are non-verbal and may be associated with psychotic spectrum disorders:

- The person may be seen shadow boxing as though fighting with someone who is not there.
- There may be a tendency for the person to stare at areas of the room where no one is present. He or she may also gesture or nod as if communicating with someone who is not there. This may be suggestive of auditory or visual hallucinations.

- The person may wear multiple layers of clothing. This may be done by an individual suffering from psychosis because they are responding to various sensations in their body which they may feel is threatening the integrity of the body. However, it is important to note that sometimes individuals with histories of living in institutions or congregate living situations may do this to protect their possessions. It may also be exhibited by individuals with developmental disabilities in response to sensory integration needs rather than suggestive of a psychotic disorder. However, this behavior may also be seen in individuals with intellectual disabilities that have been sexually or physically abused who are trying to protect themselves.
- Sometimes an individual with a psychotic disorder may try to cover their eyes or cover their ears in an effort to stop either auditory or visual hallucinations.
- The person's affect may be incongruent with what is occurring in the current situation.
- The person may be seen by others simulating a romantic or sexual interaction with a person or object which can be an indication of a tactile hallucination or a command hallucination. The individual may also be responding to flashbacks of sexual abuse during these instances. (However, there are uncommon forms of complex partial seizures that may also include sexualized auras or sexualized behaviors.)
- The individual may glare with intensity at familiar people or even strangers. This could signal paranoid delusions or it could also occur because something about that person may have triggered memories of a past abuser.
- Brushing off something that is not there may signal a tactile hallucination. However, it may also be in response to feeling some physical sensation that occurred during a traumatic event that is being re-stimulated.
- The person becomes mistrustful of people who were previously trusted. This could signal paranoia or delusions but may also be trauma induced.

Any of these behaviors may be suggestive of an underlying psychosis in an individual with an intellectual disability. However, with some of these behaviors other diagnostic caveats should be considered such as PTSD or even certain neurological conditions such as different forms of seizure activity. Sometimes the overlap of symptoms between psychosis and PTSD can make a diagnostic distinction confusing among this population. Therefore, it is important to take the time to fully assess for whether or not other PTSD criteria are present in order to make a diagnostic distinction. When evaluating for either the presence or absence of PTSD and any other co-occurring psychiatric condition(s), it is important to interpret the individual's behaviors within the context of their life histories, their other symptoms, and their health status. If the diagnostic picture continues to be somewhat confusing then a diagnostic hypothesis can be considered valid if the treatments that are introduced produce symptom relief and an improvement in the individual's quality of life.

Chapter 4

The Identification of Trauma: Methods of Assessment in Individuals with Intellectual Disabilities

CHALLENGES IN ASSESSMENT

Assessing for posttraumatic stress disorder or traumatic stress symptoms in individuals with intellectual disabilities is a challenging task. The challenges are the result of a variety of factors that include the following:

- The person may not have the verbal skills or complex vocabulary needed to discuss their traumatic memories and experiences. The measures that are currently used to assess psychiatric symptoms in the general population rely heavily on the person's ability to self-report feelings and experiences.
- The individual's challenging behaviors may be erroneously attributed to behaviors which are learned. Others may think that the person is exhibiting the behavior(s) in order to gain attention or to gain access to a preferred item, etc.
- The challenging behaviors may be attributed to the developmental disability rather than to a psychiatric condition such as PTSD. This is referred to as "diagnostic overshadowing."
- The behaviors that are exhibited may not exactly resemble the criteria specifically outlined in the DSM-5 for PTSD, since individuals with intellectual disabilities may manifest atypical symptoms of a psychiatric disorder. Their symptom presentation may be changed due to physical limitations, language limitations, developmental stages, or limited experiences and social opportunities, etc.
- There are also those individuals whose behaviors may present with subclinical presentations of PTSD.
- If the individual is non-verbal and information is sought from the person's care providers, the information may be contaminated by the caretaker's own belief system or interpretations. Therefore, behaviors may be misattributed to other motives. The assessment of trauma-based reactions may also be adversely influenced by the caretaker's experiences or frustrations with the individual.

- It may be difficult for care providers to consider that some behaviors may be trauma-based due to the emotions evoked in them. For example, a care provider may feel guilty because he or she was not able to protect the person.

Assessment Measures

Perhaps it is because of some of these challenges and more, that there is a lack of standardized assessment tools to help diagnose PTSD or traumatic responses in individuals with intellectual disabilities. (Standardized measures are tests that have withstood reliability and validity studies.) A number of tests been developed to diagnose PTSD in the general population and to assess for traumatic reactions. However, there is a lack of standardized tests to assess for this condition among the people with an intellectual disability.

Among the general population, there are assessment tools that consist of PTSD symptom severity scales. These tests assess for the presence and severity of PTSD symptoms. There are also traumatic exposure scales which are usually self-report measures which assess for exposure to either a variety of traumatic events or specific types of traumatic events. The following are some examples of assessment measures that are used for the general population:

PTSD Symptoms and Symptom Severity Scales.

These may consist of either structured clinical interviews administered by a mental health clinician or self-report measures completed by the individual. They assess for specific symptoms of PTSD. The following are some common instruments used to identify symptoms of PTSD among the general population:
- ***Clinician Administered PTSD Scale for DSM-5 (CAPS-5)***. This is a 30-item structured interview administered by a clinician. It assesses for 20 symptoms listed in the DSM-5. It enquires about the onset, the duration of symptoms, level of distress, and the severity of symptoms. It also assesses for the presence of symptoms that may warrant the additional specifier of "dissociative subtype" (Weathers et al., 2013).
- ***PTSD Checklist for DSM-5 (PCL-5)***. This is a 20–item self-report measure that assesses for the 20 symptoms listed in the DSM-5 for a diagnosis of PTSD (Blevins, Weathers, Davis, Witte, & Domino, 2015).
- ***The Impact of Events Scale – Revised***. This is a 22-item questionnaire which assesses for presence of intrusive thoughts and avoidance behaviors following stressful life events (Weiss & Marmar, 1996).

Trauma Exposure Measures.

There are a variety of assessment measures which inquire about the types of trauma an individual may have encountered. Some of the measures also assess for the degree of severity of the traumatic event. The following are examples of trauma exposure scales:
- ***Brief Trauma Questionnaire (BTQ)***. This is a brief 10-item self-report measure which is derived from the Brief Trauma Interview developed by Schnurr, Vielhauer, and Weathers (1995). The respondent notes whether or not he or she

has been exposed to a series of traumatic events which may meet the DSM-IV event criterion.
- *Trauma Assessment for Adults (TAA).* This is a self-report measure that explores different types of stressful events (Resnick, Falsetti, Kilpatrick, & Freely, 1996). The individual endorses whether or not they have had exposure to 14 different life events.
- *Trauma Events Interview (TEI).* This assesses for a trauma history by eliciting information regarding different types of traumatic events which range from sexual assault to experiencing natural disasters (Green, 1991).

While these measures have been used in the general population, they have not historically been administered (or modified) for use among individuals with intellectual disabilities. Coupled with the need for more measures to identify PTSD among this population, there is also a need to identify and address an even broader range of stress reactions which may range from acute stress disorder to various sub-threshold presentations of PTSD.

A review of the literature revealed very few assessment measures available to assist in diagnosing PTSD among individuals with intellectual disabilities. A recent measure was introduced by Hall, Jobson, and Langdon (2014) entitled, *The Impact of Event – Scale – Intellectual Disabilities (IES-IDs)*. This is a 22-item self-report screening tool developed from the *Impact of Events Scale-Revised* which is a widely used instrument to screen for PTSD in the general population. Respondents are asked to identify the traumatic event and are asked questions about their feelings and behaviors regarding the event. It can be administered to individuals with mild to moderate intellectual disabilities. Initial studies of its psychometric properties suggest it may be a useful screening tool for this population.

Another assessment measure which is available for use with individuals with intellectual disabilities is known as *The Assessment of Dual Diagnosis* (ADD). It is 79-item questionnaire developed by Matson and Bamburg (1998). However, this questionnaire was not designed solely for the assessment of posttraumatic symptoms but it has a PTSD scale. It was developed to assess for a full range of psychiatric disorders and to screen for psychopathology among individuals who are cognitively functioning within the mild to moderate range of intellectual disabilities. It has a total of 13 scales and it includes a PTSD scale. The other 12 scales include the following diagnostic categories based on the DSM-IV: Dementia, Eating Disorders, Substance Abuse, Personality Disorders, Conduct Disorder, Pervasive Developmental Disorder, Somatoform Disorders, Sexual Disorders, Depression, Mania, Anxiety, and Schizophrenia. The questionnaire is administered to the individual's care provider. In a study conducted by Matson and Bamburg (1998), the questionnaire was found to have good internal consistency and high stability across raters.

There are other tests, although few, that have been developed to assess for various psychiatric conditions among individuals with developmental disabilities. However, they have not been constructed to specifically assess for PTSD symptoms. For example, the *Glasgow Anxiety Scale for People with Intellectual Disabilities (GAS-ID)* was developed by Epsie and Mindham (2003) to assess for anxiety among individuals with mild to moderate intellectual disabilities. *The Diagnostic Assessment for the Severely Handicapped (DASH-II)* assesses for psychopathology in adults with intellectual disabilities who are cognitively functioning within the severe and profound range (Matson, Gardner, Coe, & Sovner) (1991). There is also the *Psychiatric Assessment Schedule for Adults with Developmental Disabilities Checklist (PAS-ADD-10)* (Moss et al., 1993). However, these assessment measures are not specifically designed to assess for trauma-based disorders.

In assessing for trauma or stress related disorders (such as PTSD) among individuals with intellectual disabilities, McCarthy (2001) stated that an interviewer-based assessment is an accepted method for assessing for psychopathology. This consists of an interview with the individual along with an interview with an informant. The questions assess for a range of life events along with questions which screen for the specific symptoms of PTSD.

Assessment of PTSD in Children

There are researchers who suggest that the assessment tools which are used to diagnose PTSD in children and adolescents are appropriate to administer to individuals with intellectual disabilities. Some researchers have suggested that the symptoms displayed by individuals with intellectual disabilities, who are functioning at lower developmental levels, share some of the behavioral equivalents seen among children and adolescents in the general population (Mevissen & de Jongh, 2010). The researchers who have advocated for the use of these assessment measures believe these tools may be a more appropriate match for use among some individuals with intellectual disabilities. If this approach were used, there are a variety of assessment measures for use among children and adolescents, but they have not been generally administered to individuals with intellectual disabilities. The following are some examples of both trauma exposure and symptom measures for assessing the presence of PTSD among children in the general population:

- *The Child PTSD Symptom Scale (CPSS).* This is a measure of PTSD and general symptoms (Foa, Johnson, Feeny, & Treadwell, 2001). It is a 26-item questionnaire that assesses for the presence of PTSD symptoms and their severity in children ages 8 to 18. Symptoms are also rated with regard to their frequency of occurrence.
- *Trauma Symptom Checklist for Young Children (TSCYC).* This is also a measure of symptoms, and it is completed by the child's caretaker (Briere, 2005). It is a 90-item questionnaire developed in order to assess for PTSD symptoms in children between 3 and 12 years of age.
- *Traumatic Events Screening Inventory-Revised (TESI-CRF-R).* This is a trauma exposure measure consisting of 24-items assessing for traumatic or stressful experiences among children (Ippen et al., 2002).

ASSESSMENT OF TRAUMATIC EVENTS AND TRAUMATIC EXPOSURE FOR INDIVIDUALS WITH ID

Given the lack of standardized tests to assess for PTSD, trauma, and stress-related disorders among this population, this author has developed a questionnaire designed to obtain information on exposure to traumatic or stressful events among individuals with intellectual disabilities. There is also a questionnaire presented to care providers to assess for behaviors among individuals with ID that may be symptomatic of possible trauma-induced reactions. It includes the PTSD criteria outlined in the DSM-5. The behaviors that are listed are also taken from the literature on some of the behavioral equivalents which have been highlighted as possibly being symptomatic of PTSD among individuals with ID.

The questionnaire, which asks about stressful or traumatic events, was constructed to cover a wide variety of events which individuals with ID may find stressful. It can be answered by those who know the person well, such as family members, immediate or previous caretakers, and residential staff. The questionnaire for the care providers may be presented over the course of several meetings (as needed) and should be considered as part of an ongoing assessment process. It is also helpful to interview several people among the individual's support system in order to obtain more accurate reporting. The questionnaire is meant to serve as a guideline to suggest areas that can be investigated as possible sources of stress or trauma.

When administering the questionnaire, it is important to be sensitive to the care providers' experiences in recalling some of the events. The questions do not need to be asked in one sitting, since this may prove to be overwhelming. Instead, they can be woven into conversations or interviews over a series of visits. If it appears to be too distressing to the respondent, or too overwhelming to administer, the information can be obtained in other ways such as conducting a records review, interviewing the individual, and from observations of his or her behavior. The questionnaire was designed to provide a "road map" of categories to consider. It has not been tested for statistical validity or reliability but is meant to be used as a screening tool.

Caution is advised in reviewing the questions with care providers, particularly if parents are responding to the questions. The questions may elicit feelings of guilt or remorse over events that happened to their loved ones which they were unable to foresee or prevent. In addition, some parents may also be suffering from PTSD themselves. Therefore, it is important to be sensitive while covering these areas, to proceed slowly, and to not inundate the person who is answering the questions. It is also important to ask the questions in a non-judgmental and empathetic manner when reviewing these areas. The assessment is not an investigation. It is also important to present a rationale for why the questions are being asked and to try (when possible) to develop a rapport with the care providers prior to delving into some of the areas. Answers to some of these questions may also need to be gathered through a review of available records, in addition to interviewing care providers. However, the individual with the intellectual disability, if verbal, may have also spoken about past incidents that may or may not be able to be verified by records. It is still important to note what the individual has reported (even if events are not able to be substantiated). Information should be obtained regarding the recency of the event and whether or not it was a one-time event or if the individual was exposed repeatedly to the traumatic events.

A separate questionnaire was devised for individuals with intellectual disabilities who are verbal in order to obtain information on their exposure to traumatic events. The questions in this questionnaire are constructed using an open ended format. It is comprised of fewer questions as compared to the questionnaire presented to care providers. Remember: too many closed-ended questions can lend themselves to producing an atmosphere of interrogation which would not be conducive to healing from trauma.

The questionnaire that is administered to the individual with ID is followed by another questionnaire that assesses for specific behaviors and symptoms that may suggest the presence of trauma-based response. The questionnaires may be used as part of an ongoing assessment process and assessment should be an ongoing component of a treatment plan.

Questionnaire for the Assessment of Traumatic Events among Individuals with ID

The following questions can be answered by those individuals who have supported, or are still supporting, the individual:

1. **Loss and Bereavement History**

    Relationship Losses
    a. Has the person lost an important individual due to death? If so, how long ago was the loss and how many losses has the individual sustained? Was the individual present when the person(s) died?
    b. Has the person ever lost a pet that was dear to them?
    c. Has the person lost contact with friends, peers, or staff they have liked due to either change in life situations or through conflicts, etc.?
    d. How recent have these losses been either through death or through changes in life's circumstances?
    e. Have there been any changes in the person's behavior(s) after any of these losses? If so, what were those changes?

2. **Loss of Residence/Changes in Residences**
    a. How many different residences has the person had and when did the first out-of-home placement from the family home occur?
    b. Why did he or she have to leave the home? How did he or she feel about leaving the family home and how did this move occur for the individual?
    c. How were the reasons for the moves explained?
    d. How were the moves arranged? For example, did the individual have a chance to say good-bye to the caretakers or other residents, or was the move done abruptly with no closure or ability to say good-bye?
    e. Was the person ever homeless and, if so, how long ago did this occur?
    f. Did the person's behavior(s) change as a result of any of these experiences?

3. **Other Losses**
    a. Has the person experienced any losses of property that were important to him or her? For example, did the person lose any personal property through such actions as theft, destruction by peers, or because of changes in residences?
    b. Are there any other losses that the person has experienced that may have been significant? (This includes the loss of persons, places, or things.)

4. **Health Changes**

    Accidents
    a. Has the person had any accidents or injuries? What was the nature of

those incidents? (This could include falls, car accidents, or accidently being injured by someone else.) When did the accident or accidents occur?
b. How serious was the accident or injury and has it impacted the person's day-to-day functioning?
c. If the person was in a car accident, were other people involved in the accident as well and were they injured?
d. Did the person ever witness any harm to others through any type of accidents? When did this event(s) occur?
e. Were there any changes in the person's behavior as a result of any of these events?

Medical Procedures and Hospitalizations
a. Has the individual experienced any significant changes in physical health that have impacted their quality of life or their mobility in any way? When did this happen?
b. Has the individual required sedation or restraints for any of the appointments? What types of restraints or sedation have been used and how long ago were these used?
c. Has the individual had any surgeries or any invasive medical procedures that caused the person distress? If so, when did these procedures occur? How was their recovery?
d. Were there any changes in the person's behavior after any of these events?

Psychotropic Medications and Medications for Health Conditions
a. Has the person ever taken any psychotropic medications that resulted in an allergic reaction or some type of adverse side effect? These medications could include antipsychotic medications, anti-anxiety medications, medications to treat mood disorders, and medications to treat depression or any other medical condition. How long ago did this happen and how severe were the adverse side effects?

5. **Psychiatric Hospitalizations**
   a. Does the individual have a history of any psychiatric hospitalizations?
   b. Has there been a restraint history due to presenting as a danger to self or others? Were there any injuries as a result of the restraints?

6. **Incidents of Abuse**

Physical Abuse
a. Has the person ever been physically abused? What was the nature of the incident? How severe was it and how long ago was it? Was it the result of one incident or several incidents? Who was the perpetrator? (Note: this could also be a peer.) Does the individual still have contact with the perpetrator?
b. Did the person's behaviors change after any of these incidents?

Sexual Abuse
a. Has the person ever been sexually abused or sexually mistreated? By whom and what was the nature of the incident(s) and how long ago did it occur?

    b. Were there any changes in the person's behavior(s) after the incident(s)?

Emotional Abuse

    a. Was the individual ever the victim of emotional abuse? This could include being exposed to verbal abuse, yelling, taunted and teased, called names, bulling, etc. What was the extent of the emotional abuse and how recent was the incident(s)?

Neglect

    a. Was the person ever neglected by care takers? What was the nature of the neglect? How recent and how extensive?

    b. Was there ever an impaired care provider providing care? (Impairments can occur due to physical, emotional, or psychiatric illnesses that may have made it difficult for the care taker to provide adequate care.) If so, when did this happen?

7. **Exposure to Violence**
    a. Has the person ever been exposed to violence in the form of domestic violence, school violence, or community violence? (This could include witnessing gang-related violence against others, bulling of others, or threats or physical harm towards others.) How long ago did this occur?
    b. Did the person's behavior change as a result of this exposure?

8. **Legal History**
    a. Has the person ever had any negative encounters with law enforcement? For example, this would include being arrested, questioned, handcuffed, or taken to jail or prison.

9. **Other Traumas**
    a. Are there any other events that the person either witnessed or experienced that were extremely frightening or distressing to him/her?
    b. Has the individual ever been in a situation in which they feared for their safety?

Questionnaire of Traumatic Events for the Individual with ID

These questions are presented personally to the individual who is verbal and whose cognitive functioning lies within the mild or moderate range of intellectual disability. The questionnaire is constructed of open ended questions with the intention of obtaining information regarding stressful events that the person may have experienced. However, it shouldn't be presented until enough time has been spent with the individual to develop a rapport. Sometimes the individual may not trust the person asking the questions and may respond with, "Why do you want to know?" or the person may just "shut down." It is important to reassure them. Let them know that you are trying to understand what they have been through so you can help them find what can make them feel happy and safe. Trust can be an issue for a person who has undergone trauma, and the person may not trust what you are going to do with the information, so they should be aware of why you are asking the questions. Marich (2014) has noted that the *"what"* and the *"how"* questions are the most ideal for conducting trauma-informed assessments. This allows the individual to provide the amount of detail that they are comfortable disclosing at the time. Again, as with the questionnaire for care providers, the questions can be presented over time as the individual becomes more comfortable in disclosing information. Although obtaining a trauma history is important, it cannot be over emphasized that this needs to be done at a pace and at an intensity that is safe for the individual.

The following are some questions which can be presented directly to the individual:
1. Tell me about the places where you have lived. How did you like those places?
2. What was the best place that you ever lived?
3. Tell me about your family. What are your mom and dad like? What are your brothers and sisters like?
4. How do you like going to doctors' appointments?
5. Has anyone ever hit you or hurt you?
6. Has anyone ever touched you in a way that made you feel bad, angry, or uncomfortable?
7. What do you think of the medications you are taking?
8. Do you have trouble sleeping?
9. Do you ever have any bad dreams or nightmares?
10. Have you ever met any police officers? What happened when you met them?
11. Tell me about any people that you miss who you wish you could see.
12. Has anyone you loved died?
13. Have you ever fallen or hurt yourself? Have you ever been in a car accident?
14. What things make you sad?
15. What things make you angry?
16. What makes you happy?

These questions are not as extensive as the questions that can be presented to the care providers. What I have found over the years is that when asked these basic questions clients will often elaborate and begin to discuss traumatic incidents or very stressful experiences. For example, when I asked a young woman about whether or not she liked her last group home, she said that the people were "mean." She was asked to describe what they did when they were "mean," and she said the staff would yell at her and the other clients would throw things and hit people when they were mad. When I have asked clients to tell about the best place that they have lived they will usually talk about what they liked about the staff and the activities in the home as well as the other residents. For example, one individual said that the staff were very nice and talked to him "a lot" and took him out shopping and out to eat. If the individual said he or she did not like living in a particular group home, they will usually elaborate on what they didn't like. There have been many times when the individual stated they wanted to live with their parents and not in any group home. This can also provide information on attachment histories and major disruptions in those attachments.

The questions are also aimed at assessing whether or not the individual has had any encounters with the law. Such experiences may have been the result of the person acting in a dangerous manner necessitating police intervention. This could have led to experiences with involuntary hospitalizations or even an arrest which can be traumatic.

Since nightmares and sleep disturbances can be hallmark symptoms of PTSD (Matsakis, 1994), there are two questions regarding the individual's sleeping and whether or not they have bad dreams. However, it is also important to note that sometimes psychotropic medications can cause bad dreams and insomnia. Therefore, it is important to ensure positive endorsements to these questions are not reflective of medication side effects. There is also a question about going to the doctor in order to assess for any experiences with medical appointments that caused fear (i.e., invasive exams or procedures, etc.).

As part of the assessment, it is important to also look for themes or trends. If the individual is reluctant to answer the questions, it is important to not force the situation. Trauma-informed or trauma-sensitive interventions avoid introducing situations or demands that may re-traumatize the person. If a person is not comfortable talking about the situations, continuing to push for disclosure can add to their distress. Safety and flexibility are two key components to being trauma-sensitive in interactions. The person may not yet feel safe to disclose information, and trust may need to be established first. Therefore, screening for trauma may be a process that gradually unveils information until the full picture is understood. Sometimes, even with time the person may be fearful to disclose problems in the past for fear he/she will be blamed for what had occurred. The person may be used to people focusing on their behaviors rather than focusing on the underlying motivations for those behaviors.

All too often individuals with intellectual disabilities have been the victims of many forms of abuse in their lives, and they have never been asked about their experiences. If you ask, be sure that you are not leaving them with open emotional wounds and with no methods to cope.

It is important to also be sensitive to the fact that some individuals with intellectual disabilities will answer the questions even if they are not comfortable because they have been taught that it is unacceptable to say "no" or they may want to please. Therefore, it is important to also watch for any non-verbal signs of agitation during questioning. If you start to see agitation, stop the questioning or give the person permission to stop. It is important to be flexible. The information can be gathered at another time or through other avenues (i.e., interview with care providers, review of records, direct observation of behavior, etc.).

As with the questions provided to the care providers, it is important to provide a rationale for your questions and to explain how the information will be used. Otherwise, you may encounter a response such as, "Why are you asking me?" The person may fear he or she is in trouble or something may happen to him/her if they tell the truth. However, there is also the possibility that the person may exaggerate or fabricate answers in order to get someone in trouble. Again, looking for themes, obtaining information from various sources, and getting to know the person will help to ensure greater accuracy.

It is also important to consider the family system and cultural aspects of the person's experience and to be sensitive to these areas. For example, there was a situation in which a mother and her developmentally delayed son immigrated to the United States from another country. The young man and his mother suffered both emotional and physical abuse at the hands of the father. However, the mother did not leave for fear that he would be granted custody which was the custom and law in her country if a woman leaves her husband. Consequently, the abuse did not end until the father died. Such a family situation was extremely difficult for the client's mother, as well as for her son, and both needed time to heal. In such situations, proceed with caution and sensitivity and above all try to do no harm.

Possible Trauma-Related or Trauma-Induced Behaviors

In addition to obtaining information from the care providers and the individual (when possible) regarding the occurrence of stressful or traumatic events, the assessment process should also take into consideration behavioral presentations that may suggest possible trauma-based reactions. Obtaining information regarding behaviors is particularly important in trying to assess for trauma-related reactions in individuals who are non-verbal and whose cognitive functioning may be in the severe and profound range of intellectual disabilities. In assessing for traumatic stress reactions and indicators of PTSD among this population, it is helpful to obtain information regarding behavioral challenges that may reflect some of the symptoms found in the four symptom clusters used to diagnosis PTSD.

Avoidance Behaviors
1. Does the person avoid any environments? If so, what types of environments does he/she avoid? How long has this been occurring?
2. Does the person avoid interacting with certain people? If so, are there specific characteristics of those individuals that seem to bother the individual?
3. Does the individual avoid certain activities? What types of activities does he/she want to avoid by resisting participation?
4. Did any of these avoidance patterns start after something happened in that environment or after something happened to that individual? Was there a delay in exhibiting the behavior from the time of the stressful event or traumatic event?

Alterations in Arousal and Reactivity
1. Does the individual excessively or repeatedly scan the environment? Does the individual keep exploring the environment, as if looking for any signs of danger?
2. Does the person startle easily?
3. Does the person have problems falling asleep or staying asleep?
4. Is the person physically aggressive towards others? Are there any commonalities in the people that are the targets of assault (e.g., tall men)?
5. Does the aggression seem to occur "out-of-the-blue?"
6. Does the person have angry outbursts that are sometimes exhibited with little provocation?
7. Does the individual have any addictive behaviors (e.g., food, drug or alcohol abuse, or sexual addictions)? (The presence of addictive behaviors such as compulsive gambling, compulsive overeating, or engaging in self-injurious behavior may also be maladaptive methods used to decrease the level of arousal experienced in the nervous system.)
8. Does the person engage in any behaviors that are self-harming such as self-injurious behavior (e.g., head banging, biting oneself, hitting oneself against hard surfaces, etc.)? Does the person take any objects and engage in self-mutilating behaviors?
9. Is the person physically aggressive towards others?
10. Does the aggression often come "out-of-the-blue?"

Marked Alterations in Cognition and Mood
1. Does the person ever have instances in which he/she shuts down or detaches from interactions and may become non-responsive or socially withdrawn? Under what circumstances does this occur?
2. If verbal, has the individual ever discussed experiencing difficulties trusting people?
3. If non-verbal, does the individual appear to need a prolonged period of time before they seem to be comfortable with new people? Is the person ever aggressive towards unfamiliar people?
4. Does the individual ever show signs of happiness or positive emotions (e.g., smiling, laughing, etc.)?

Intrusive Symptoms
1. Does the person exhibit any signs of agitation upon awakening that could suggest bad dreams or nightmares?
2. Does the individual exhibit periods of distress or agitation under certain circumstances? What are those circumstances? Are those circumstances similar to the traumatic situation the person experienced?
3. If the person is verbal, has he or she ever discussed memories of past traumatic or stressful events to indicate that he/she is still actively thinking about these events?

When viewing some of these behaviors it is also important to be aware of other possible diagnostic caveats that could account for them. Some common alternative explanations among this population are as follows:
- An exaggerated startle response may be more reflective of sensory sensitivities in the individual based on the developmental disability, such as what can occur in autism. It is also possible that some of these sensory sensitivities could be misinterpreted as heightened arousal suggestive of PTSD. This may also occur in someone who is losing their hearing.
- Aggression can sometimes occur in those individuals who are losing some of their sensory capabilities such as decreased sight or hearing. This can occur particularly in those individuals with severe and profound intellectual disabilities whose eyesight is failing due to cataracts.
- Sometimes the sensory stimulation that occurs in some environments may be overwhelming to individuals with intellectual disabilities. This can result in agitated behavior, and sometimes even aggression, as they try to indicate a need to escape the situation.
- Some of these behaviors such as social withdrawal and persistent negative emotions such as increased irritability may be attributable to another psychiatric condition such as depression.
- Sometimes medication side effects can affect sleep and even produce vivid dreams or nightmares. Therefore, it is important to look at a medication time line to ensure that these behaviors are not better attributable to medication changes.

- Sleep issues may also occur more frequently in individuals who have more severe levels of an intellectual disability.
- It is always important to rule out any possible medical conditions that may mimic psychiatric conditions or result in an acute onset of behavioral challenges or an increase in existing behavioral challenges.

HISTORY TAKING AND GETTING TO KNOW THE INDIVIDUAL

What cannot be emphasized enough is the need to get to know the individual and his or her history. This is particularly important when working with individuals with intellectual disabilities who are non-verbal, but it is also very important in working with individuals who are verbal. Gathering information about their lives is important in trying to identify any events that may produce PTSD symptoms or trauma-like reactions. Constructing a time line of events in an individual's life, and changes in behavior as a result, can provide clues to whether or not PTSD, or even partial PTSD, may be present. Interviewing previous caretakers, family members, and support staff and mining through any available records are important ways to uncovering past stressful events or trauma. Gathering observational data is also important. Direct observations become particularly important when the individuals are non-verbal and cannot describe their internal experiences.

In assessing for the presence of PTSD, or even the presence of subthreshold PTSD symptoms, it is important to remember that behaviors that are reflective of traumatic reactions generally result in a change in the individual's baseline level of functioning. However, the diagnostic process can become more challenging when the PTSD is chronic and based on events that occurred many years ago. Therefore, it is important to look at the chronology of symptoms. What were the behaviors like prior to the traumatic or stressful events and what have the behaviors been like since the event(s)? If the traumatic or stressful events were not recent, how long ago were they and did the behaviors change for either a short period of time after the event or have the behavioral changes been long-standing? What supports and treatments were offered after the traumatic event(s)? Although gathering this information may be a time-consuming process, consider the time involved when these dynamics surrounding trauma are not properly identified and treated. How many care provider hours and consultant hours may have been invested in trying to address behavioral challenges without successful results? Consider the valuable time lost that could have been invested in providing the proper treatments. More importantly, consider the time lost for the individual by not having a better quality of life.

Chapter 5

Trauma-Informed Treatment and Trauma-Informed Care

The concept of providing trauma-informed care (TIC) is an approach that has been evolving over the past few decades. As an understanding of the pervasiveness of trauma, and its relationship to a variety of physical, behavioral, and emotional disorders has grown, service delivery systems have become more responsive to the needs of individuals impacted by trauma. As reported by Fallot and Harris (2009):

> Trauma can be fundamentally life altering, especially for those individuals who have faced repeated and prolonged abuse and especially when the violence is perpetrated by those who were supposed to be caretakers. Physical, sexual, and emotional violence become central realities around which profound neurobiological and psychosocial adaptations occur...Trauma may shape a person's way of being in the world; it can deflate the spirit and trample the soul. (p.1)

This awareness has led to the developmental of evidence-based models of treating trauma which have also included changes not only in the types of services that are delivered but also changes in the administrative and organizational structures of the agencies providing those services.

Trauma-informed care is an approach that recognizes the widespread impact trauma can have on a victim's life. It is grounded in an understanding of the neurobiological, psychological, physical, and social impact trauma can produce. The primary goals of trauma-informed care include the identification and recognition of trauma-related symptoms, training of support personnel in the impact of trauma, the avoidance of any re-traumatizing approaches, and the education of institutions or service agencies to ensure they do not inadvertently re-enact the dynamics of trauma (Harris & Fallot, 2001; Hodas, 2006). A trauma-informed approach incorporates several basic principles:

1. ***Recognition*** – It recognizes the impact that traumatic experiences can have on individuals and the paths that are needed to facilitate recovery. It understands the widespread impact that trauma can have and how treatments may be ineffective if the impact of trauma is not recognized or treated.

2. ***Safety*** – Trauma-informed care recognizes that the need to feel safe is an important part of recovery and healing from trauma. It emphasizes both physical and emotional safety. This approach seeks to educate organizations and

individuals about the dynamics of trauma so that support personnel do not operate in ways that may inadvertently re-traumatize the individual.
3. ***Collaboration and Mutuality*** – It recognizes the need to ensure that the people who are supported have a "voice and choice" in their recovery. It helps to empower the person.
4. ***Cultural Sensitivity and Responsiveness*** – Such an approach remains cognizant of cultural factors and gender issues and remains sensitive to understanding these differences. When people feel understood, it sets the stage for greater collaboration and a sense of equity. The meanings attached to trauma may vary depending upon cultural variables among cultures, and individual responses may also vary across cultures.
5. ***Dependability and Compassion*** – A trauma-informed approach helps to promote dependable and compassionate relationships which can facilitate healing.
6. ***Resiliency*** – There is a focus on rebuilding an individual's strengths and introducing factors that can promote resiliency and healing.

Trauma-informed care has found its way into a variety of different service delivery systems. Its principles and accompanying interventions are being introduced into the foster care system, the educational system, health care systems, alcohol and drug treatment programs, the juvenile justice system, and in the behavioral health arena. If these systems, and the people working within them, understand trauma and its impact, it can help to facilitate a more compassionate and well-informed approach. It can reduce the likelihood of introducing interventions that are ineffective because they do not appreciate the complexities and the pervasive impact caused by trauma. Understanding a person's life experiences and how trauma has played a role increases the potential for greater patient engagement and cooperation with treatment, as well as enhancing staff and provider wellness.

Systems that do not operate utilizing a trauma-informed approach have increased risks of pathologizing the behaviors of the people they serve. The focus becomes one of identifying what is wrong with the person rather than focusing on understanding what has happened to the individual. There can also be a misuse of power, and the system can become coercive and controlling. The organization itself, if it doesn't apply some of the same principles to the employees who provide the service, can suffer a higher turnover of staff and decreased morale among staff.

Since individuals with intellectual disabilities have higher prevalence rates of abuse than the general population, and are in many ways a more vulnerable population due to the nature of their disabilities, incorporating a trauma-informed approach is a much needed focus. It is important that care providers or anyone supporting individuals with developmental disabilities use the principles set forth in trauma-informed care. It is important to help ensure the environments that individuals with intellectual disabilities are exposed to promote physical and emotional safety. It is also important that consistent and healthy boundaries are established and maintained by those who support them. It is important to help restore a sense of control and predictability to the lives of people impacted by trauma. Trust also becomes a significant issue. Individuals with PTSD and trauma-based reactions may have difficulty trusting others. Therefore, the development and maintenance of dependable, transparent, and consistent relationships becomes an important part of healing. There also needs to be a focus on building individuals' strengths, improving their social support systems, and introducing the factors that promote resiliency. Utilizing a trauma-sensitive or trauma-informed approach can also help care providers, parents, and clinicians to be more vigilant in considering whether or not some of the behavioral challenges, psychiatric symptoms, and/or physical complaints exhibited by the individuals they support may be trauma related. This will help to ensure that individuals with intellectual disabilities and trauma histories receive the appropriate treatments.

In order to ensure a more trauma-informed and trauma-sensitive workforce, individuals who support people with intellectual disabilities should possess the following information:

- Agency staff as well as care providers should be aware of the many different types of trauma facing this population. This should include even more hidden or covert forms of abuse. They should be aware of the different types of trauma-based reactions which can occur. Consequently, when they see these behaviors occurring or medical conditions occurring, it may prompt them to further investigate the underlying causes.
- Individuals providing supports and services for this population, whether in the role of a direct care professional or a clinician from a social service agency, should receive training on the impact that culture, race, gender, age, sexual orientation, and socioeconomic status can have on experiences of trauma (Jennings, 2004).
- Training on trauma should also include information regarding its prevalence among this population and the fact that there is individual variability in the evaluation and experience of what constitutes a traumatic event. Therefore, it is important to avoid judging whether or not a person with an intellectual disability has experienced trauma by one's own standards.
- In supporting individuals with developmental disabilities, think "trauma first." When trying to understand why a person is behaving the way they are, it is important to consider the possibility that they may have been the victim of trauma. The person's behaviors may be in response to traumatic events. Review the individual's history. Are there any known incidents of abuse or violence? What types of situations has the person endured that may have been traumatic?
- Consistent relationships characterized by healthy boundaries facilitate healing in individuals who have experienced trauma. Therefore, training in how to establish and maintain healthy boundaries is important for all who serve this population.

With regard to the concept of consistency, if the person experiences a high rate of turnover among support staff, which could include social workers as well as direct line staff, it can be very disruptive. Therefore, it is important to have community residences, as well as human service agencies, that have low turnover in staff. Studies have been conducted that have examined the variables that impact longevity of employment and found that providing adequate monetary compensation, appropriate vacation leave, and ensuring employees feel supported by their employers are important factors which decrease staff turnover (Hoge et al., 2007). In order to facilitate staff retention in agencies that support individuals with trauma histories, it is also important that workloads are kept at manageable levels and job roles are well defined. Having a competent and cohesive team of co-workers is also very important.

The same factors that facilitate healing in the people they serve should also be introduced at an agency's administrative level. Ideally, trauma-informed approaches should also be incorporated into an organization's operating policies and mission statements.

Specific Trainings in Trauma-Sensitive Interventions

In order to create safety, both at an emotional and physical level, and to incorporate the principles of trauma informed care, the following are some specific strategies for use by both direct care staff and administrators who support individuals with intellectual disabilities. It is important that trauma-informed services and approaches are incorporated into staff development trainings and into administrative practices. The interventions that are suggested are more general in nature. They are not a substitute for seeking professional assistance in order to develop trauma-focused assessments and interventions that utilize specific therapies and techniques.

Strategies for Administrators and Managers of Adult Residential Facilities

When operating a residential home or facility that serves individuals with intellectual disabilities with trauma histories, it is particularly important to establish a safe environment in the home. Creating such an environment includes ensuring that staff members are trauma trained and sensitive to the issues created by trauma. The following are recommended strategies that can be used to promote healing and safety in the residence:

- Consider the mix of personalities of the clients you have agreed to support in your facility/residence. If a client in your home has a history of being physically abused, having them live with someone who has a significant history of aggression towards peers can reactivate past traumas and hinder healing.
- Be informed about the history of the individual you are supporting. What was the nature of the trauma they experienced? Was it abuse by a certain person? If so, does the client person still react negatively to individuals with similar characteristics? For example, if the client was emotionally abused by a tall red haired woman, avoid staffing the shifts with a person of similar physical description or characteristics. By knowing the trauma triggers for the individual, this will provide clues regarding the best way to staff the home.
- It is very important that the staff understand the client's trauma triggers so they can understand why the person may react the way he or she does. It is important to try and remove as many of those environmental or interpersonal triggers as possible, or minimize them.
- Ensure the staff are well trained in the person's history prior to the individual's admission to the home. If the staff are not familiar with the person's history, to include the individual's behavioral challenges and any history of trauma, staff may inadvertently act in a way that could re-traumatize the individual.
- It is important that staff are familiar with the situational triggers for the challenging behaviors of the individuals they are supporting. Staff should be

trained in the most effective way to prevent the behaviors prior to the individual's admission.
- Staff should receive training in de-escalation strategies and crisis communication. This should include training in active listening techniques. This will help to diffuse situations before behaviors escalate.
- It is important to have a crisis support plan in place for the staff to follow if none of the de-escalation strategies are effective. The staff need to know what to do in the "worst case behavioral scenario." This will help them to feel safer. However, if the behavioral crises are frequent this usually means that the individual's support plan is not effective and should be re-evaluated.
- It is important for the staff to have a working knowledge of the individual's stress-related symptoms. How does the individual react when they are under stress? Does the individual react emotionally, behaviorally, or physically, or through a combination of any of these? It is important to incorporate stress reduction techniques for the client into the support plans.
- It is important to have proper staffing ratios to intervene quickly for those individuals who have significant behavioral challenges. This will also help to lessen the stress on the staff.
- Ensure that staff maintain good boundaries and therapeutic relationships with very clear roles. Staff training in how to maintain professional relationships is important. This will also facilitate healing as the clients know what to expect. This will help to ensure that their relationships remain consistent and predictable which facilitates the development of trust. Establishing healthy boundaries includes ensuring that physical, emotional, and financial boundaries are effectively set. It is important for the staff to remember that they are not the resident's friend, or substitute parental figure, or therapist. The staff are important support individuals in that person's life, and the nature of their relationship should be therapeutic.
- It is important to create an environment that respects the individual's dignity. This is the client's home. Maintain their surroundings in a manner that conveys respect and caring.
- Create a physical environment that is conducive to healing.
- Clients should be informed of their rights as well as their responsibilities.
- Since control is often taken away in tragedy and trauma, it is important to try and provide the individuals you support with choices in their lives whenever possible. This can help to promote a sense of control over their environment. When emphasizing choices and responsibilities, do so using language that is clear, concrete, and simple.
- If behavioral consultants are providing consultation services, it is important that their assessments routinely screen for histories of trauma and trauma-related symptoms and behaviors among the residents. Trauma histories and their impact should be considered in constructing any behavior intervention plans.
- It is also important to consider environmental factors and how to help establish a sense of safety. Consideration should be given to how to create a sense of safety in congregate living situations. The homes should be large enough

or have private bedrooms or areas, such as patio areas where the clients can retreat if peers are exhibiting any disruptive behaviors. Disruptive behaviors may include screaming, yelling, property destruction, or aggression. These behaviors directed towards peers and/or staff can create anxiety in the other residents which can make them feel unsafe. It is also important to have staff reassure other clients in the home that they are safe and will be protected if peers are acting out.

- Ensure in the interview process that you are hiring people with good boundaries (e.g., good physical and emotional boundaries). Part of establishing good boundaries is also ensuring that the staff are able to be fair but firm in setting limits with the individual.
- It is also important that the staff are consistent both in their attendance and in their interactions with the clients. If there is a high staff turnover, it can be very unsettling for an individual with a trauma history, since trust may be difficult for the client to establish. If relationships are consistent and dependable, it can help to re-establish trusting connections. Therefore, it is important to hire staff who are committed to being consistent in their work attendance. However, this may require higher monetary compensation or other employee benefits in order to ensure lower staff turnover. When hiring employees, here are a few words of wisdom that were posted once in a human service's agency by an anonymous author: "Hire your people with care and care for the people you hire."
- Consider the gender of the staff you are hiring in relation to the types of trauma experienced by the clients.
- Trainings should also include self-management and stress management strategies for staff, given the level of stress than can accompany working with individuals with trauma histories.
- Being trained in the principles and concepts of trauma-informed care, or even basic behavior management strategies, does not necessarily ensure their day-to-day implementation by direct care staff. Therefore, it is recommended that there be supervisory or administrative support to ensure these concepts are applied. Supervisory support has also been shown in studies to lessen the stress on direct support professionals (Stanley et al., 2010). Spend time in your facility.
- Ensure you have a psychiatrist who is a member of the individual's support team along with a behavioral consultant and a mental health provider. Clinical staff should also have received training in trauma-sensitive approaches and strategies. The collaborative and comprehensive approach that an interdisciplinary treatment team offers allows for the whole person to be considered in the development of a treatment plan and the delivery of services. Facilitate and encourage a team approach.
- It is also important to consider the mix of personalities in the people that are hired. Working collaboratively as a team can lessen the stress on the job and improve job performance (Ford & Honnor, 2000; Snow, Swan, Raghavan, Connell, & Kelin, 2003).
- It is important that staff receive adequate instruction in order to do their jobs

and that their job descriptions are well defined. There is research regarding work stress among direct support professionals which has indicated that role confusion can lead to increased stress on the job and increased stress can increase the risk of depression among workers.
- In creating a trauma-sensitive organization and a trauma-informed workforce, it is important to ensure collaborative efforts occur between the various community agencies providing supports. This can be particularly challenging or difficult if the agencies themselves are inadvertently acting in ways that can re-traumatize the very people they are serving. To the best of your ability, advocate for the client.
- Provide ongoing training in trauma-informed care for direct support professionals. Provide the rationale to the staff for incorporating trauma-informed services.
- Obtain feedback from the residents about the services that are being delivered.
- Ensure your facility has a disaster plan. Since you are serving individuals with trauma histories, be proactive in reducing the impact that future traumatic events may have. This would include developing a plan for service provision should a disaster strike (e.g., earthquake, fire, storms, etc.). Plans should also include how to protect clients' records in the case of an evacuation. It is important to identify high risk clients who would be psychologically impacted to a greater extent, given their histories. Identify what specialty services they may need post-disaster.
- It is important to ensure that the services and supports being provided to the client are linguistically responsive. Communication is very important. It is important for the client to be able to communicate to the staff if they are verbal. For example, if the client is deaf but uses American Sign Language (ASL), then it is important that staff are also trained in ASL. If the client is non-verbal, it is important for the staff to understand how that individual communicates. This information may be obtained from individuals who have worked closest with the person or who have the best working knowledge.
- Pay attention to conflicts among residents in the home. It may not be enough to just separate them. Inadequately resolved conflicts among residents can also trigger a trauma response in some people depending upon their histories. Help resolve the issues or take steps to modify or eliminate the problem.
- If meetings are periodically scheduled to review the client's treatment plan and progress, be sensitive to the way in which the meeting is convened and the way the information is presented to the client. It is important to ensure that the format of the meeting does not re-traumatize the individual. Some clients find it very anxiety producing to have to attend meetings in which there are a number of staff present, including clinicians, who are going to talk about their behaviors, their medical conditions, and personal information, etc. The way the client's meetings are structured should be evaluated on a case-by-case basis. The format for including the individual, obtaining his or her input, and providing feedback to the person should be designed in a way that promotes healing and removes or minimizes any trauma triggers. For example, the cli-

ent may only want to meet with a few trusted staff and not an entire team. This may be less threatening. The entire interdisciplinary team can still convene, but the information should be conveyed, and any input obtained from the client, in the least anxiety provoking manner. It is all too often that clients are forced to attend their meetings when no one has given them the opportunity to decline participating. With clients who are non-verbal, their behaviors may reflect either their willingness to attend or their desire to refuse and those wishes need to be considered. For example, if a non-verbal client is escorted to a large meeting and upon entering the room assaults the person next to her, the environment may be too threatening or over stimulating. Remember that safety and choice are very important components of trauma-sensitive interventions. However, this may be in direct opposition to an agency's usual standard operating procedures. Again, this is why trauma informed care also promotes trauma-sensitive approaches at the organizational level.

- Upon admitting a new client to a community residence/facility, it is not uncommon to hear care providers asking family members to wait a month before visiting. Some care providers have adopted this philosophy as a means to help the client adjust to the new home and lessen confusion. It is recommended that this philosophy, if used, be re-evaluated on a case-by-case basis. Otherwise, it runs the risk of re-stimulating issues related to any history of separation, loss, or disrupted attachments. Consider how you would feel if you just moved into a new place, changed jobs, were now surrounded by new people, new things, etc., and were told that you could not see the people important in your life for one month. Social support has been one of the factors which has repeatedly been shown to lessen stress. Again, it is recommended that this philosophy not be incorporated as a blanket facility policy but evaluated on a case-by-case basis. If there are concerns about possibly confusing the client by having the family visit, it may be best to talk with the client's family before admission to discuss the most appropriate way to arrange visits or contact. If the individual's family members are important supporters of the resident, maintaining regular contact with them is also recommended. Discuss with them what they need to do to be able to support the person in the best way possible. If their contact is detrimental to the individual, then other measures or interventions may need to be created with the help of the individual's social worker or other supporting professionals.
- Keep lines of communication open with both your staff and your clients.
- Provide a stimulating home environment that includes opportunities to access the activities and leisure skills that the client enjoys.
- Decorate the home with consideration for the individual's behavioral challenges or any sensory impairments. For example, if a client has been known to throw objects when mad, avoid decorating with glass or objects that can be easily thrown and shatter, etc.
- Help clients increase their safe coping skills.
- Staff should be well versed and trained in the warning signs of abuse and neglect for individuals with intellectual disabilities as well as reporting obligations.

- As an administrator for a residential facility, providing a stable environment that is predictable, with healthy boundaries established by the staff, and consistent limits, can help the client learn new skills and promote recovery. However, it is critical to ensure that you have hired appropriate staff for the job and that they are specifically trained in trauma-based strategies.

Strategies for Group Home or Adult Residential Facility Staff

The following are general strategies recommended for use by direct line staff who support this population:

- Avoid a style of interacting that is controlling or authoritarian in nature. This is likely to produce a negative effect. Again, control is an important theme for someone who has been the victim of trauma. Limits, boundaries, and consequences can be established for challenging behaviors, but they can be delivered in a firm but calm manner. They should not be delivered in a coercive or controlling manner.
- Communication and the style of communication are important. When supporting individuals with trauma histories, an interpersonal style of respectfulness, trustworthiness, and consistency helps to facilitate healing.
- If the client is in distress, use the client's best skills to help them calm down. This may include such activities as talking, drawing, throwing a basketball, or other ways they can use to discharge their tension, self-soothe, and find safety. If the client is verbal, it may be helpful to ask, "What can you do to feel better or what can we do to help you feel better?"
- It is important to model how to appropriately express emotions in ways that maintain a safe environment.
- Avoid delivering any consequences for behavior in a punishing manner with anger.
- If the individual has aggressive behavior which occurs "out of the blue," note the details leading up to the situation. For example, did a particular staff member approach the client with a certain tone of voice? Was the approach rapid? This may help provide clues to identifying any trauma triggers that may be occurring. Aggression occurring "out-of-the blue" can sometimes be an indication that something has just triggered a traumatic memory in the individual which produced the overreaction.
- A multi-disciplinary or treatment team approach is important especially in working with someone with a trauma history and an intellectual disability. When supporting individuals with significant behavioral challenges, and both mental health issues and intellectual disabilities, it is important to be able to rely on your co-workers, as well as collaborate with clinicians who should also be part of the team.
- Be aware of the individual's trauma history and any trauma triggers they may have so that trauma triggers can be avoided.
- Maintain professional boundaries. You can be warm and friendly but still maintain appropriate boundaries. There are a variety of ways that boundaries can become too diffuse or enmeshed and not well established. These include

some of the following: taking too much of a personal interest in the client and performing tasks that are outside of normal job duties specifically for that person, sharing personal information that is not needed for the person's growth or well-being, providing home phone numbers so the client can contact you, or becoming defensive around any issues with the client. An example of crossing financial boundaries would be borrowing or lending of money to a client.

- Provide choices for the individual whenever possible. This will help the individual to re-establish a sense of control over his or her life. However, for some people being confronted with too many choices can be overwhelming.
- It is important to refrain from acting in ways that may re-traumatize the individual. Avoid the use of coercive techniques and avoid forcing agendas. Such interventions can result in the unintentional re-traumatization of the individual.
- Remember the importance of social support in mitigating stress. Help facilitate the development of a healthy support system for the person.
- Identify the activities that are self-soothing to each resident so that when he/she is upset or under stress, you can encourage them to engage in these activities or make the activities available. Introduce stress reducing activities in the home so that their home becomes a safe and healing one.
- Help to ensure their sense of safety. If there is another client in the home whose behavior becomes threatening to other residents, ensure those residents feel safe and protected. If another resident's behaviors begin to escalate, ensure that staff who are not immediately dealing with the situation are cognizant of the reactions of the other residents and are attending to them. This may involve reassuring them or redirecting them to a quieter place in the home or encouraging them to go to their rooms to relax.
- If a client with PTSD does not appear to be responding to the events in the "here and now" but may be having a flashback, grounding techniques can be helpful. This would involve orienting the client to what is happening in the present. Get them to focus on something that is happening in the current moment.
- Identify the strengths of the clients and their coping skills. Ensure that the activities that are scheduled help to build the individual's leisure skills and enjoyment. Such leisure skills or hobbies can also help to build the person's sense of accomplishment. Unstructured time can be an invitation for more behavioral challenges.
- When supporting individuals with challenging behaviors, including emotional outbursts and physical aggression, it is helpful to create safe zones or spaces in the home. Since some of the higher level group homes are meant to serve individuals with these behavioral profiles, it may not be possible to avoid having someone with a trauma history living with someone who exhibits these behaviors. If this is the case, it is important to help them feel as safe as possible. For example, letting them have a private bedroom can be helpful. They can escape to the privacy and solitude of their own space if they feel threatened. If another peer in the home is acting out, perhaps he/she can go out into the community to escape the chaos provided there is enough staff available. Hav-

- ing staff nearby to also reassure the individual that they are safe and no harm will come to them can be comforting.
- It is also important to change aspects of the environment that may feel threatening to the client. For example, if the client has a history of being assaulted at night by another resident, avoid placing their bed in a position in the room in which they can't see who is coming in the room.
- Do not judge whether or not the person may be traumatized based on your own interpretation or reaction to the situation. Each person is different, and an event that may traumatize one person may not have the same reaction in another.
- Be vigilant for any evidence of abuse and report it. Don't ignore it or rationalize it away.
- Be aware of any fearful reactions or avoidance behaviors the resident may exhibit which may suggest a traumatic experience. For example, if a resident comes home from the day program and then suddenly refuses to use the bathroom, explore all possibilities for changes in behavior (e.g., medical, psychiatric, or the possibility of abuse which may have occurred in a restroom, etc.). Consider the possibility of the avoidance response being trauma-based.
- For individuals who startle easily, avoid approaching them rapidly. The startle response can be a symptom of PTSD.
- Be well versed and trained in de-escalation strategies. When an individual with a trauma history is triggered, he or she may be responding out of past memories and experiences rather than correctly evaluating the reality of the "here and now." Pay attention to any signs of distress in the client, intervene early, and assess for any unmet needs. Try to redirect behavior if it is escalating by providing some reasonable choices or options for another activity or course of action.
- When working with an agitated client, ensure his or her safety, the safety of the other residents, your own safety, and the safety of the other staff. Watch your own body language so as to avoid any gestures which can be misconstrued as threatening. Monitor what is in the immediate environment to ensure nothing can be used by the client as a weapon. Do not allow yourself to be cornered. Be vigilant of your surroundings. Avoid any coercive approach and avoid threatening the individual with a consequence for his or her behavior, since this may escalate the situation. Try to help the individual manage their distress and emotions and regain control. If the individual is verbal, ask them what they need to help the situation.
- Working with an agitated client requires a team effort in order to maintain everyone's safety. Know the whereabouts of your colleagues as a situation starts to escalate. Ensure the physical space is arranged for safety.

Strategies for Parents

As a parent, if your son or daughter has suffered some form of trauma, the following are some guidelines to facilitate healing:
- Get back to establishing a routine at home. Establishing consistent and predictable routines and daily patterns is important in lessening anxiety and fostering a sense of safety.

- If your son or daughter is isolating him- or herself from other people, schedule some pleasant and fun activities. Provide some positive experiences, but the fun activities should not include any items or circumstances that could remind them of the traumatic events.
- It is a natural reaction to want to protect your child after a traumatic event. However, overprotection to the extent that you are reinforcing avoidance and withdrawal is not going to be helpful. If your child or adult child is afraid to go somewhere as a result of the trauma, gradually and very slowly exposing him/her to aspects of the situation he/she has been avoiding can help lessen the fear. Avoidance reactions do not often go away on their own (unless the person is really motivated to confront the situation) but get reinforced because of the reduction in anxiety they can produce.
- Be vigilant and watchful for signs of posttraumatic symptoms such as sleep difficulties and avoidance behaviors. Note the situations in which these symptoms occur. If your child or adult child is exhibiting any of the symptoms, it is possible that they encountered some type of trauma trigger that reminded them of the past stressful events. Being vigilant to these cues may help you to remove any trauma triggers in the environment in the future.
- Provide choices whenever possible. These can also be forced choices. For example, you can ask, "Would you rather take a shower before or after your television show?" You can even frame consequences using a choice format.
- Provide reassurance and nurturance. Assure your son or daughter that they are safe.
- Expectations for behaviors and rules and consequences still need to be applied. Use positive reinforcement for desired behaviors.
- If your child or adult child with ID is confused and is trying to understand what happened, provide explanations that are simple, clear, and appropriate for the individual's developmental level.
- Manage your own stress level.
- Educate yourself so that you know what to expect and what are some typical reactions to trauma. Learn about the factors that promote resiliency.
- Be patient. Healing takes time, and recovery is not always linear.
- Help your child to learn to manage overwhelming emotions. Help him/her to identify some self-soothing activities that are calming. If the emotions become too overwhelming and lead to severe behavioral melt-downs, this may require professional help and support.

CARE FOR THE CARETAKER

Part of adopting a trauma-informed perspective also involves considering the people who provide the service. It would be remiss to talk about the topic of identifying and treating trauma among individuals with intellectual disabilities without discussing the topic of traumatic-like reactions and stress responses among care providers (i.e., family members, friends, foster parents, etc.). Although being a caretaker can be very rewarding, it can also be very overwhelming.

With regard to parents who are the care providers and other first degree relatives, this writer has met numerous families throughout the years, in the course of providing behavioral consultations, who are exhausted, overwhelmed, and exhibiting trauma-like responses themselves. These stress reactions can occur in response to the hardships and stress they encounter supporting their young children and adult children with developmental disabilities.

The stress that care providers may experience can lead to physical symptoms, behaviors, and psychiatric symptoms that can simulate a type of posttraumatic stress reaction. Perhaps, the reactions may not be exactly the same as if the individual was involved in a horrific or tragic event, but nonetheless, their reactions may have similarities. Their symptoms, behaviors, and experiences may not meet the criteria for a diagnosis of PTSD, but they may be experiencing similar symptoms. In an article entitled, "Caregiver PTSD: Fact or Fiction" by Ann Napoletan (2013), she states that although PTSD has been usually associated with soldiers and combat and horrific events, the impact and emotional upheaval that can occur with being a caregiver can provide its own source of trauma which may produce some symptoms representing a form of PTSD.

Families of individuals with developmental disabilities are often tasked to provide frequent and sometimes constant care and supervision, depending on the exact nature of their family member's disability. For example, there are numerous syndromes which can cause intellectual disabilities and have medical correlates to the syndrome as well. Consequently, care providers may continue to face periodic health crises with their loved ones. Some of the medical issues are even chronic and progress with time. If behavioral challenges or psychiatric issues are also added to the scenario, they may leave the care provider in a constant state of having to be hypervigilant.

Sometimes behavioral challenges necessitate a constant level of monitoring in order to either prevent their occurrence or to ensure the behaviors do not escalate to a crisis level. This can be particularly stressful as in the case of potentially harmful behaviors such as self-injurious behaviors or aggressive behaviors. It can be emotionally and physically taxing for caretakers to have to support individuals with behaviors which can pose a danger to the person themselves or to others. Anger and a sense of helplessness and hopelessness may follow. Families may feel isolated in their battles to gain an understanding of their loved one's behaviors and how to manage or prevent them. They may be living in what can feel like a battle zone because they never know what the day is going to hold, and if the individual is going to attack them or injure him- or herself.

Over the years, this author has heard some parents discuss feeling as though they are being held hostage in their own homes. They are fearful of taking the individual out in the community or to certain places in the community for fear he or she will act out and will cause a scene in public or someone may get hurt.

This author has also talked with parents who are so deeply distressed by their son or daughter's self-injurious behavior that it has been overwhelming for them. They feel helpless to stop the person from hurting themselves. I recall one parent describing her morning when she walked into her adult daughter's bedroom to wake her up. Her daughter was non-ambulatory with cerebral palsy and an intellectual disability in the moderate range. Her daughter had been compulsively biting her hands and picking at her wounds. When her mother opened the door to wake her up she found her daughter awake already. Her mother stated, "There was blood everywhere." This was the first night her mother had tried to sleep in a separate bed. She had been sleeping with her daughter so that she could try to prevent her from harming herself at night, since this behavior had begun to resurface. The young woman's mother was exhausted and needed a good night's sleep, and this was what she encountered upon awakening. The stress can be enormous on families when managing severe self-injurious behavior or aggressive behavior.

In a small study conducted by Hodgetts, Zwaigenbaum, and Nicholas (2015), researchers interviewed family members who were living with individuals with autism who were aggressive. Eight families participated in the study, and the authors identified "three central processes." The families experienced financial stress and limited supports. According to the authors, there was a detrimental impact on the families' daily routines as well as having adverse effects on the well-being of family members. From their research, they found the families to be exhausted, isolated, and in need of more services such as respite. They had to live with frequent concerns for their own safety and well-being. The families in their study also experienced limited professional assistance.

Another study conducted by Seltzer et al. (2009) at the University of Wisconsin-Madison also studied the experiences of a group of mothers of adolescents and adults with autism over the course of eight days. They interviewed the mothers at the end of each of the eight days, and hormone levels from the mothers were drawn on four of the days to assess their stress levels. According to their findings, it was discovered that a hormone that is associated with stress had low levels, and the levels were consistent with military personnel who had served in combat.

The study also found that the mothers in their research spent on the average of at least two additional hours per day providing care for their children as compared to mothers of children without disabilities.

Additional stress may be experienced by families of individuals with intellectual disabilities if psychiatric issues are present in addition to behavioral challenges, and in some cases in addition to medical conditions. Supporting individuals who are also dually diagnosed (i.e., have a psychiatric disability and an intellectual disability) can present with unique challenges. If the psychiatric disorder is contributing to behavioral challenges, it can be a complex, confusing, and highly stressful situation for care providers. The sources of care provider stress in these types of situations can include a lack of sleep and not being able to meet with friends and connect with their own support systems. There is also the added burden of potential financial difficulties. The care provides may not be able to work outside the home due to their responsibilities as a caretaker. If the stress experienced by the care provider remains chronic with little or no remittance, it can lead to burnout which can be problematic for both the care provider and the person in their care.

Care Provider Stress and Burnout

If the responsibilities for caring for someone with a disability are not managed well, they can become a source of chronic and accumulating stress resulting in an increased risk for depression, anxiety, and physical symptoms. Chronic stress and multiple stressors can lead to burnout in time, if the stress is not alleviated or managed well. Stress and burnout are linked but they are not the same. Burnout does not occur without being initiated by stress but stress doesn't always lead to burnout. It only leads to burnout if it continues to accumulate and worsen. However, there are negative consequences to health and psychological well-being of stress and burnout, particularly if stress remains chronic.

According to Pines and Aronson (1988), burnout involves a state of physical exhaustion as well as emotional and mental fatigue. This can occur as a result of being in very emotionally demanding environments for extended periods of time. Some of the signs and symptoms of burnout can simulate the symptoms of PTSD and can include feelings of hopelessness and helplessness, apathy, and blunted affect. The person experiencing burnout may also be plagued with intrusive thoughts that also involve mental representations or pictures of the struggles encountered by the people being supported whether those struggles consist of psychiatric, behavioral, or health related crises.

Self-Care Plans

Working with individuals who have dual diagnoses (i.e., intellectual disabilities and psychiatric disorders such as PTSD), or who exhibit some type of trauma-based reactions, necessitates a good self-care plan whether you are a family member, staff, or clinician. It is not easy for the care providers who provide the daily care for these individuals and for the staff and clinicians who do trauma-based work. It can take its toll, perhaps not with the same intensity of first-line responders who are in the throes of rescuing individuals from life or death situations, but nonetheless, it has it owns stressors. For example, consider the foster mother who cares for developmentally disabled abused children. I am reminded of a colleague, a social worker, who once told me she had been providing foster care for an infant who had suffered brain damage from being beaten by her biological mother. She cared for the infant to the best of her ability. She would soothe the infant who would cry frequently and who was blind because of the abuse. She did this because she loved children and out of the goodness of heart and with the best of intentions. However, she was mandated to return the baby to the biological parents after a court hearing. It was the court's desire for the family to be reunited within a short period of time. She had to respond to the court order to return the child not knowing if the child would suffer again at the hands of her biological parents. She felt helplessness and powerlessness. She cried for a day or two until another call came in asking her to provide foster care for yet another infant. She didn't have time to cry any longer. She had to move on. She had to regain her focus and let go of what she couldn't control. This can be a difficult path to traverse and providing care under such difficult circumstances can be stressful.

Consider those individuals with intellectual disabilities whose trauma-based reactions include aggression, non-compliance, anger outbursts, or self-destructive behaviors. Imagine the stress on families or staff as they try to evade punches and attacks and try to de-escalate potentially escalating situations. This stress can be compounded by working within systems that are not trauma- sensitive or are unable to provide sufficient resources due to budgetary constraints. Consequently, it is important for care providers (i.e., parents, staff, foster parents, etc.) to be aware of their own symptoms of stress, since each person's reactions to stress are as unique as their fingerprints. Some people will exhibit mostly behavioral symptoms when stressed, some will exhibit physical symptoms, and others will exhibit emotional symptoms. Some people will experience a combination of symptoms from several of these categories. It is important for care providers to map out their own unique symptoms that indicate that their stress levels are increasing. It is important to pay attention to these early warning signs so that the accumulation of stress does not progress into burnout.

When developing a self-care plan it is best to have a plan that is comprehensive. In theory, a holistic approach to self-care would address several different areas and include a plan for emotional self-care, as well as physical, spiritual, and psychological self-care. Spiritual can be a broad category that is not limited to only religious activities. This can include simply engaging in activities that have personal meaning or provide the individual with a higher sense of purpose.

The following are some suggested strategies to promote self-care and protect against burnout while supporting individuals with trauma histories:

- *It is important to spend time with people in your support system.*
  When people are stressed sometimes they tend to withdrawal and isolate. It is important to connect with the people you care about and with the people who care about you. This helps to provide a balance in life. Throughout the stress management literature, social support has been repeatedly identified as a mitigator of stress.

- *Know your limits.*
  It is very important to know your physical and emotional limits. I have seen care providers take on too much out of compassion and out of a sense of duty and obligation. For example, it can be very difficult to remain patient and understanding when supporting a family member with an intellectual disability who has mental health issues and exhibits dangerous behaviors. Group home administrators may want to help out of compassion by accepting someone for admission into their home when in actuality, they may not have sufficient staffing or staff who are experienced enough. By exceeding one's own limits, resources, capabilities, etc., the best of intentions can go wrong and sometimes produce tragic results.

- *Get a good night's sleep.*
  The importance of getting a good night's sleep cannot be overemphasized. Sleep deprivation can compromise an individual's health and emotional well-being.

- *Maintain a balanced life-style.*
  It is important in discussing self-care to emphasize the need to maintain a balanced life style. This can be the most challenging tasks and one of the most critical. In the book by Covey (1989) entitled *The 7 Habits of Effective People*, he identified the principle of "sharpening the saw." He used the analogy that if someone chops down trees repeatedly the saw will eventually become dull. The work will become harder and an individual's efforts less efficient because of the worn out saw blades. Taking time to rest and replenish leads to greater efficiency. Also, without the time to recharge, a care provider's quality of care can become compromised.

- *Develop self-soothing rituals or activities.*
  It is important to develop self-soothing rituals. These should consist of healthy and positive self-regulating activities and not ones that are potentially self-defeating such as drinking too much or habitually overeating. Take a bath. Take a walk. Listen to music. Find those activities that are not potentially harmful.
- *Develop a daily structure and organization to your life.*
  When stress is chronic, there is sometimes a breakdown in an individual's daily structure and routine. This can happen when people feel overwhelmed and tired. Unfortunately, this can increase the stress in the home for both the care provider and the person being supported, if the person lives in that environment. Chaotic or unstructured environments can trigger behavioral challenges in some individuals with intellectual disabilities. A lack of structure and predictability can lead to greater anxiety and increased stress. Routines can provide comfort and reduce stress.
- *Reconnect or connect with positive experiences.*
  When working under stressful conditions it is important to take time to connect with positive experiences in life. This is especially true when working with trauma. It is important to balance the negative with positive experiences. It is important to connect with life and the better parts of it which are not associated with abuse, tragedy, loss, etc., but are more reflective of life's joys. For example, spend time with a friend who has a young baby. Take a walk along the beach and enjoy the beauty that nature has to offer. People involved in trauma work need to be reminded to experience the joys of life as a way to balance the tragedies of life. There needs to be a balance in life between the positive and the negative.
- *Exercise.*
  Tension and stress impact the body, and the tension needs to be discharged. Taking a walk, working out, riding a bike, or any form of exercise can improve both mood and your physical health. Spend time with nature. Go hiking. Go to the mountains or to the beach.
- *Connect with activities that provide a higher purpose.*
  Since spirituality is a personalized area of someone's life, determine what spirituality means to you. Does it equate with religion or a faith? If so, cultivate those areas. If not, find other areas or avenues that call you to a higher purpose in life. For example, volunteer to help in a homeless shelter around the holidays.
- *Develop surrender skills.*
  Developing surrender skills is a main tenet of stress management. Learn to let go of what you cannot control.
- *Address family conflicts constructively.*
  When managing care giver stress among when the care is being provided by family members, it is important to identify and address any family conflicts that may be related to providing care. When family members are the providers of most or all of the care they need to develop rotating schedules and take time off.

- *Maintain good nutrition.*
  Eat healthy. Make a commitment to maintaining healthy eating habits.

TRAUMA-INFORMED SYSTEMS

A trauma- informed approach is meant to extend to not only the direct care providers or the professionals, it is also meant to address the systems that provide the supports and services. When a system is working within the framework of being trauma-sensitive, it seeks to avoid any interventions that may serve as triggers for trauma or may inadvertently re-traumatize the individual. For example, consider the case of an individual with a developmental disability in the mild range of cognitive functioning who has had numerous disruptions in her attachment history. She had to leave her family home as a young child and move into a residential facility. After the move her parents stopped coming to see her, and then they passed away. She moved from group home to group home due to a variety of reasons including her challenging behaviors, as well as a care provider closing one of the homes. She was eventually admitted to a crisis center for short-term treatment and stabilization. Her length of stay was mandated by the law and state regulations. Within six to nine months she had to move to another location because of regulations. Her behaviors just began to stabilize with consistent staff and staff who provided a safe and positive environment. Then she moved to another facility that has a high staff turnover. Consequently, she continued to encounter frequent disruptions in her relationships. No sooner did she become used to staff and even start trusting them, then they would leave or she had to change facilities or residences. Year after year this continued, and her behavioral challenges escalated until she was rejected by a number of different care providers and entered into what seems to be a perpetual cycle of psychiatric hospitalizations and discharges. There was no consistency, no sense of safety or predictability, which are some of the factors that can promote healing.

Consider another scenario in which an individual with a mild to moderate level of intellectual disability and psychiatric issues, along with behavioral challenges, moves into an adult residential facility. Numerous clinical supports are provided along with an enhanced staffing ratio. Under these circumstances, the individual begins to flourish. His behaviors improve along with his psychiatric symptoms because of the additional supports and interventions. The individual has a significant trauma history which has consisted of physical and sexual abuse by relatives while living at home and by peers while living in various placements. This is the first time in his life that he has been in a predictable, structured environment with consistent staff and he starts to feel safe. His personality is also compatible with the three other individuals who live in the home. However, one of the other residents moves to another state with his family leaving one opening in the group home. Social workers from the agency want to admit another individual to the home from a nearby psychiatric facility. There are no other homes with openings that have this level of augmented services for that particular individual. The clinicians at the psychiatric hospital do not feel they can make any further progress with him, since their hospital milieu is not designed to support individuals with intellectual disabilities. However, the individual can still be aggressive towards staff and peers, but he no longer meets the criteria for admission since he is not presenting as an imminent danger to others or to himself. He is admitted into the home and he begins to be physically aggressive towards all the individuals in the home including the resident with the trauma history. In response to these events, the individual who had been doing well starts to regress both behaviorally and psychiatrically.

These scenarios are all too familiar and the result of systems that are not trauma sensitive either due to a lack of training, resources, budgetary constraints, or regulations, etc. It is important to examine the systems that serve individuals with trauma histories and to advocate and challenge aspects of the system that hinder healing. Regulations and policies can have an impact on a person's recovery. Consequently, introducing a trauma sensitive approach may require a paradigm shift within the systems supporting individuals with intellectual disabilities and trauma histories. As Marich (2014) aptly noted, one of the major problems with addressing and treating trauma in today's professional service environment is that agencies, to include hospitals, often adopt a "one size fits all" approach. Adopting a more individualized approach may be considered by agencies to be too time-consuming and costly. Often when clients do not conform or improve within the treatment standards being offered by that agency, they may be labeled as being resistant to change and/or not motivated to make any changes. This mode of operating needs to be changed if agencies want to adopt a trauma-informed system of care in clinical arenas.

Chapter 6

Risks and Resiliency

Not everyone who is exposed to trauma and tragedy becomes traumatized. Upon review of the statistics regarding the prevalence rates of PTSD among individuals exposed to trauma and tragedy, it is evident that many people are resilient. According to Frans, Rimmo, Aberg, and Fredrikson (2005), only 8% to 12% of the individuals in the general population exposed to trauma develop symptoms severe enough to warrant a diagnosis of posttraumatic stress disorder. Helzer, Robins, and McEvoy (1987) quoted statistics that were higher and found that 20% to 30% of people who were exposed to trauma in the general population developed symptoms severe enough to warrant the diagnosis with a life-time prevalence rate of 9.2% whereas studies which have explored the prevalence rate of PTSD among individuals with intellectual disabilities have quoted figures ranging from 2.5% to 60% (Firth et al., 2001; Wigham, Taylor, & Hatton, 2014). Some studies have also indicated that lower developmental levels are associated with a greater risk of developing PTSD and developing more severe symptoms (Macklin et al., 1998; McNally & Shin, 1995). Given the wider range, the risks would appear to be higher for individuals with intellectual disabilities. So, what variables increase the risk of developing PTSD, and what factors serve as protective mechanisms against its development? If these factors have been identified in the general population, do the same variables apply to individuals with intellectual disabilities?

The search for factors that may increase an individual's risk of developing PTSD began early in the history of identifying posttraumatic stress disorder. Since not all individuals exposed to traumatic events develop symptoms severe enough to warrant a PTSD diagnosis, researchers began looking for other factors responsible for its development rather than simple exposure.

One of the first systematic studies which investigated the risk factors for developing PTSD was conducted by Foy, Sipprelle, Rueger, & Carroll (1984). In that study it was discovered that an important factor which predicted the development of PTSD was the nature or the extent of the exposure to the traumatic event. A dose response relationship between the severity of the exposure and the development of PTSD was also found by other researchers (Halligan & Yehuda, 2000). However, subsequent studies have found that only a small portion of the variance in PTSD was accounted for by the characteristics of the traumatic event (Breslau et al., 1998). Researchers began to identify a variety of other variables that predicted the development of the disorder.

These risk factors can be divided into three different categories: pre-traumatic, traumatic, and post-traumatic factors. The following are factors which have been identified in each of these categories as risks for developing the disorder:

PRE-TRAUMATIC FACTORS

1. *Previous traumatic experiences early in life make one more susceptible.* If trauma is experienced very early in life (particularly in the form of childhood neglect, abuse, or abandonment), it can increase the risk of developing PTSD. Stovall-McClough and Cloitre (2006) reported that individuals with unresolved childhood trauma have a seven times greater risk of developing PTSD than those without this type of childhood history.
2. *A history of trauma is predictive.* Prior trauma (or traumas) which resulted in a previous diagnosis of PTSD may make someone more susceptible to future reoccurrences of the disorder (Schiraldi, 2000).
3. *A lack of coping skills makes one vulnerable.* Individuals who suffer from low self-esteem, who lack problem-solving abilities, and who are more emotional are more vulnerable to developing PTSD (Schiraldi, 2000).
4. *Age is predictive.* An individual's age can be a factor. Younger individuals are more vulnerable to developing the disorder than their older counterparts. Friedman (2000) noted that individuals younger than 25 were more likely to develop PTSD than their older counterparts.
5. *High levels of stress in everyday life makes a difference.* If an individual has had recent stressful events in his or her life, it can weaken psychological defenses again trauma induced stress (Schiraldi, 2000).
6. *Gender is a risk factor.* Being female has been identified as being a risk factor for PTSD, but it has also been identified as a risk factor for the development of other psychiatric disorders (Breslau, Chilcoat, Kessler, Peterson, & Lucia, 1999). Since females have an increased risk of experiencing interpersonal violence (particularly sexual violence), some speculate that this may be the factor or factors contributing to its development. Studies have found that sexual violence results in higher rates of PTSD (Kimerling, Ouimette, & Wolfe 2002). Some studies have shown that although men may experience more traumatic events in their lifetimes than women, women are more likely to develop PTSD (Perkonigg, Kessler, Storz, & Wittchen, 2000). Not only are women at an increased risk to develop the disorder but their symptoms tend to be more chronic (Kimerling et al., 2002).
7. *Having biological family members who have PTSD or who have been diagnosed with other mental health issues makes one more vulnerable.* Researchers have found that individuals whose biological parents or first-degree relatives suffered from anxiety disorders, mood disorders, and substance abuse disorders were more likely to develop PTSD (Durand & Barlow, 2006).
8. *There are biological vulnerabilities.* Some people may have more of a biological propensity to respond to trauma with an overactive nervous system. They remain genetically more vulnerable to the impact of stress and trauma (Gilbertson et al., 2002).

9. *Having other mental health issues such as depression and anxiety increases the possibility of PTSD.* Researchers have found that PTSD is more likely to occur among those individuals who suffer from co-existing psychiatric disorders such as substance abuse, depressive disorders, somatization disorder, and anxiety disorders (Keller et al., 2006; Kessler et al., 1995; Mills, Teesson, Ross, & Peters, 2006).
10. *There are cognitive risk factors.* Studies have shown that an individual's level of cognitive/intellectual functioning is a risk factor for the development of PTSD. In an early study by Macklin et al. (1998), the researchers assessed the IQ scores of soldiers prior to entering battle. Having made an adjustment in the study for the degree of exposure to battle, they found that individuals with lower IQ scores had an increased risk of developing PTSD. Studies have already shown an increased risk of all psychiatric disorders among individuals with intellectual disabilities. Prevalence rates of psychiatric disorders among individuals with developmental disabilities have varied depending upon differences in sampling, classification, and screening. Some studies have quoted prevalence rates ranging from 15.7% (Cooper et al., 2007) to 54% (Gustafsson & Sonnander, 2004).

PERI-TRAUMATIC FACTORS

1. *Proximity to the trauma is predictive.* The closer someone is in physical proximity to a traumatic event, the more likely he/she is to experience greater distress and a greater likelihood of developing PTSD (Pynoos, Frederick, Nade, Arroyo, & Steinberg, 1987).
2. *The nature of the trauma may affect the rate of PTSD.* Certain types of trauma are more likely to produce PTSD than others. For example, trauma that is the result of interpersonal violence is more likely to lead to PTSD than trauma experienced from a natural disaster. Vulnerability to developing PTSD increases when the trauma is unexpected, reoccurring, sudden, or chronic (Schiraldi, 2000).
3. *Experiencing intense trauma or long-lasting trauma (i.e., duration of the exposure and severity) may lead to PTSD.* The greater the magnitude of the trauma, the more likely it is to result in PTSD (Durand & Barlow, 2006).

POST-TRAUMATIC FACTORS

1. *A lack of social support makes one more vulnerable.* Poor social support can be a post-traumatic risk factor, since social support has been a variable that is pervasive in the literature for helping to mitigating stress. Consequently, if someone has a poor social support system, it may increase the likelihood of developing PTSD.
2. *A lack of treatment affects the outcome.* A lack of treatment for PTSD itself may lead to chronic symptoms (Kessler et al., 1995).
3. *Secondary victimization may occur.* This occurs when the individual is re-traumatized by those who are supposed to be supporting or helping the victim (Schiraldi, 2000).

Predictor Variables for PTSD among Individuals with ID

From the list of factors that may predispose an individual to develop PTSD in the general population, it becomes clear that no single factor is responsible. There are a variety of psychosocial variables and genetic, and environmental factors which may all contribute. Although researchers have identified these variables among the general population, there has been a lack of systematic studies on the factors which increase the risk (as well as the factors which mitigate the risk) of developing PTSD among individuals with intellectual disabilities. Given the lack of such systematic investigations, we are left with reviewing predictor variables among the general population and extrapolating and hypothesizing that some of these factors may also have applicability to individuals with intellectual disabilities.

In this author's experience, several factors have emerged throughout several decades of work with this population that appear to increase the risk of developing PTSD or partial PTSD. However, these factors have been based solely on anecdotal and clinical experiences and not on a systematic study of predictor variables. One of the factors which have surfaced repeatedly among individuals with ID (who are verbal) is the trauma associated with having been removed from their families of origin at a young age. It has been this author's experience that some of the individuals with the most challenging behaviors (and numerous psychiatric disorders) have had numerous disruptions in their early attachment histories. Such histories have included separation either due to loss, neglect, or abuse by their biological parents. In some cases, these early disruptions in their attachments have been followed by placements in which peers have either been violent towards them or have sexually abused them. As a result, some of these individuals have had the greatest difficulty in regulating their emotions, and they have often had extensive psychiatric histories with numerous psychiatric diagnoses and hospitalizations.

RESILIENCY

The concept of resiliency spans many areas and disciplines with a variety of definitions. In its most general and simplest form, resiliency refers to a person's ability to adapt to stress or trauma by returning to a healthy level of psychological and physical functioning (Daniel, 2007; Tugate & Fredrickson, 2004). It refers to an individual's ability to recover and adapt well after experiencing significant stress or adversity. Other terms that have been closely related to this concept have been words such as "hardiness," "resourcefulness," "learned optimism," and "adaptive coping."

Psychological studies of "resilient" people have identified several characteristics and external factors which contribute to an individual's resiliency. Several studies have explored the factors which promote resiliency in adults as well as in children. In studies of children who have experienced overwhelming stress, researchers found the following factors foster resiliency:

- *Self-esteem* – The individual has a good sense of self and self-worth. They know what they like and dislike, and they feel valued (Hyman, Gold, & Cott, 2003).
- *Support systems* – The child has a good social support system and has individuals he or she can rely on for comfort and support (Hoge, Austin, & Pollack, 2007).

- *A sense of belonging or affiliation* – The child feels connected to a supportive group, whether it be a church or a volunteer group. There is a sense of belonging and connection (Hyman et al., 2003).
- *Autonomy* – The child feels as though he or she has some control over what happens in his or her life.
- *Positive experiences* – There are positive experiences with people outside the stressful environment (Hyman et al., 2003).

Researchers who have studied resiliency in adults with regard to PTSD and stressful events have identified several factors which not only promote recovery from exposure to trauma and stress but also serve as protective factors against the development of PTSD. Some of these factors include:

- *Good coping skills and an active coping style* – Individuals who are good at problem-solving and regulating or managing their emotions fair better. These are active problem-solvers who can also accept their emotions, identify them, and regulate them (Park & Adler, 2003).
- *Social support* – A significant mediating variable for promoting well-being that is found extensively in both the stress and trauma literature is having a good social support system which includes resilient role models (Resick, 2001).
- *Moral compass* – Individuals who are resilient tend to have a strong set of morals and principles which guide them. Altruism is one way to facilitate resiliency. Helping others can result in a sense of fulfillment (Hagland, Cooper, Southwick, & Charney, 2007).
- *Cognitive flexibility* – Individuals who can cognitively reframe or reappraise situations from negative to positive are more resilient. According to neuroimaging studies, individuals who use cognitive appraisal and reappraisal strategies have a greater ability to deal with adversity. They have a "top-down" control of their emotional reactions. By engaging in cognitive reappraisals, they activate the prefrontal cortex of the brain which helps to regulate the limbic symptom which is the part of the brain responsible for emotions (Hagland et al., 2007; Ochsner et al., 2004).
- *Positive self-concept* – Individuals who are confident in their abilities, their talents, and their strengths, fared better.
- *Regular physical exercise* – Engaging in physical exercise helps to support physical health as well as to improve mood. It helps to lessen the negative emotions that can be caused by stress (Hagland et al., 2007).
- *Maintaining a positive outlook* – Maintaining one's sense of humor and viewing adversity as more of a temporary condition, rather than a permanent or pervasive one, are important ways to promote a more positive outlook and to avoid pessimism (Hagland et al., 2007).

Promoting Resiliency from Trauma and Stressful Events among Individuals with Intellectual Disabilities

By the very nature of their disability, individuals with intellectual disabilities have had their resiliency tested to a much greater extent than the general population. They have had to learn to cope not only with cognitive limitations but often with other limitations brought about by their developmental disabilities (e.g., physical, social, or speech, etc.). Such challenges require a level of adaptation and coping. If trauma, tragedy, and stress are then added into the equation, imagine the greater challenges these present to their resiliency skills.

Despite the obstacles and adversities individuals with intellectual disabilities face (as well as the increased prevalence of trauma in this population), there is a lack of studies on the construct of resiliency as it applies to individuals with intellectual disabilities. The research literature exploring the variables that promote resiliency and serve as protective factors in the general population is significantly more prolific. Consequently, we are left to take these findings and extrapolate and modify them for application with this population. Since individuals with intellectual disabilities are a separate at-risk population for experiencing trauma, improving strategies for promoting resiliency should be an important focus.

The following are suggestions for resiliency-promoting interventions for individuals with intellectual disabilities as adaptions from the existing literature:

- Improve their coping skills by teaching and promoting problem-solving skills. This could be done by providing the concrete steps that comprise this skill. This also helps to improve the individual's executive functioning skills which are important in regulating emotions (Greenberg, 2006).
- Help them foster positive relationships. Teach them the skills needed to develop and maintain friendships and nurture their existing relationships.
- Foster their personal interests so that they can experience greater fulfillment in life. Often individuals with intellectual disabilities have few developed leisure skills or hobbies. Often, unstructured time and boredom can be an invitation for behavioral challenges.
- Help them to maintain optimism and hope. Trauma can make people lose hope, see only a dim future ahead, and sometimes even see a foreshortened future. Helping to provide hope and creating events and things to look forward to can inspire positive feelings.
- Foster social affiliations so that they can experience a sense of belonging. For example, helping a person to connect with a church or a volunteer organization can help promote a sense of identification, belongingness, and self-worth.
- Look at what strengths are present, and acknowledge them, and encourage greater development of those strengths. Help encourage and promote their talents in realistic ways.
- Help promote a sense of self-sufficiency. Whenever possible, help them build their skills so that they may have greater independence and a sense of autonomy. This could be as simple as helping a person learn how to cook (if this is appropriate given the individual's level of cognitive functioning). Help the individual to feel more competent, and to feel as though they can affect positive change in their life. It is important to help them establish goals that are realistic and goals that can be realized over time by creating steps needed to attain the goal.
- Help promote social activities and social competencies. Studies have shown that individuals who are functioning within the mild range of intellectual

functioning experience less severe anxiety if they are socially active (Corray & Bakala, 2005). This may also help them to build trust which might have been shattered by the traumatic experiences.
- Surround them with positive people. Individuals with intellectual disabilities can sometimes be sensitive to the anxieties of others surrounding them.
- By their very nature transitions involve change and change can equate to stress. Promote efforts to better facilitate transitions since traumatized individuals can sometimes be very sensitive to transitions. Help ease their anxieties surrounding change by helping them to know what will happen and what they can expect in advance of the event. This can be accomplished through the use of pictures, visual schedules, and verbal reassurances. Use multiple ways to present the information. Introduce transitions gradually and with time to prepare for the event whenever possible.

Neuroplasticity and PTSD Recovery

Developments in the field of neuroplasticity indicate the human brain is able to heal and even rewire itself after trauma. In the past, it was thought that our brains were fixed and that change in its structure was not possible as people reached adulthood. However, research during the past few decades has indicated that our brains are, in fact, able to create new neural pathways and produce new neurons (Doidge, 2015). These neural pathways become strengthened with repetition. Years ago, a Canadian psychologist, Hebb, suggested that when two neurons fire at the same time they start to connect. This actually can lead to changes in the structure of the brain. "The neurons that fire together, wire together" (Hebb, 1949). Therefore, if an individual continues to have a repetition of an experience it can lead to actual changes in the brain or, more specifically, the way the neurons process that information in the brain. The neurons will have greater connections with consistent experiences. By repeating something in a focused manner, new neural pathways are developed. Over time, these pathways become so familiar that they are easily accessed as a default mode by the brain.

What does this mean for people in the general population who suffer from PTSD? It means that the brain is capable of changing if people are committed to recovery and committed to putting experiences in their lives that can change these neuronal connections. The brain can change with different experiences. Rewiring the brain to release fear and replacing experiences with those geared towards introducing safety and control can facilitate recovery. An example of Hebbian theory would be if an individual reacted to any minor failure in his or her life with a self-statement of self-loathing and worthlessness, and did this repeatedly, then there would a neural pathway that associates setbacks or failures with a sense of worthlessness. This association would eventually become an almost effortless and automatic process for the person. However, if the person began to challenges this association when confronted with any setbacks or failure by making a statement such as, "I am a capable person" and did so whenever faced with the same situation, a new neural pathway could be established. Initially, the individual may not believe this thought was authentic because the association is weak at first. It would take repetition of this association before a new neural association is forged.

What could these findings mean for individuals with intellectual disabilities? If Hebb's theory that neurons that "fire together, wire together" is considered for this population, it would suggest that individuals who support them must make a concentrated effort to help them change their experiences and introduce new positive experiences. Although negative, traumatic experiences can change people, positive experiences geared towards introducing safety and the maintenance of positive social attachments may help the recovery process. Therefore, it means that the people who support them must help make these new experiences and positive connections possible for them, and they must help to ensure that the traumatic experiences do not keep reoccurring. It is also important to help them form more positive identities and not identifies forged by a handicap. Individuals with intellectual disabilities and trauma histories need to be in healing and safe environments with social connections that promote positive, consistent, and safe attachments. With Hebbian theory in mind, such positive experiences may be able to promote the creation of new neural pathways for healing.

Chapter 7

Treatment of Traumatic Reactions in Individuals with ID

When is treatment for trauma needed? If the effects of the traumatic experiences do not dissipate with time, and the person has not returned to his or her previous level of functioning, treatment should be considered. If the individual is experiencing significant disturbances or impairments in his or her ability to function as a result of the event or events, treatment should be obtained.

Experiencing trauma can cause disruptions in someone's physiological, psychological, and social functioning. Recovery from trauma takes time, and it does not occur in a neat, linear fashion. Treatment involves a series of phases including stabilization, integration, and adaptation. Initially, it is important to acknowledge the traumatic event and its impact on the individual. During the early phase of stabilization, it is important for the individual to develop an ability to self-regulate. Treatment then can progress to a phase of integration during which trauma arousal diminishes and a sense of safety begins to be restored. During the phase of adaptation, the person starts to reconnect with the world. Consequently, the treatment of trauma involves helping the individual gain control of his or her emotions, restore resiliency, and restore the person's sense of safety and control. From a neurobiological perspective, treatment should also involve re-establishing a balance in the individual's nervous system in order to decrease symptoms of hyperarousal. If the autonomic nervous system remains out of balance, with the sympathetic nervous system remaining dominant, the individual is more likely to act impulsively and without self-reflection. This could lead to self-destructive behaviors, interpersonal difficulties, emotional reactivity, and even addictive behaviors. This physiological imbalance could also erode an individual's physical health. Therefore, it becomes important to help regulate a dysregulated nervous system.

There are a variety of treatments used in the general population to treat posttraumatic stress disorder and specific methods for treating different types of trauma. Several of these treatments are also used in treating individuals with intellectual disabilities who suffer from PTSD or even sub-threshold PTSD. However, regardless of the type of treatment approach that is used to treat PTSD, there are a number of common goals among these various therapeutic approaches, both for use with the general population and among individuals with intellectual disabilities. Interventions are geared towards decreasing the symptoms of hypervigilance or hyperarousal, reducing intrusive memories, and reducing social withdrawal and avoidance reactions. Treatments help to re-establish an individual's basic needs. These needs include the need to be connected to others, the ability to trust in others, to feel safe in the world, to feel valued, and to feel some sense of control in life (Rosenbloom & Williams, 1999). If these needs were to be prioritized, it is this author's belief and professional experience that the need to feel safe, the need to trust, and the need to have some control over one's life are the most critical elements to re-establish in working with individuals with intellectual disabilities. Although the need to feel valued and connected is also important, the first three elements geared towards establishing safety and trust are the most essential, particularly when working with individuals whose cognitive levels of functioning lie within the lower ranges (e.g., severe and profound). As Rosenbloom and Williams (1999) noted, the dimension of safety includes the need to feel safe with yourself, to feel safe with other people, and to feel safe in the world.

Being Safe with Oneself

When addressing the need for individuals with intellectual disabilities to feel safe with themselves, consider the fact that negative emotions can be very overwhelming. Such emotions can feel very uncomfortable and potentially dangerous to the individual. It brings to mind the interview this author once had with an individual with mild ID who was morbidly obese and would compulsively overeat. In addition, he would also injure himself whenever he felt a strong emotion. He would insert sharp objects into various orifices in his body when he was angry, sad, or lonely or when he experienced some other negative emotion. He had a trauma history of parental abandonment, and he also lived in poverty with relatives who were homeless and living on the streets with him. The police became involved, various agencies came to assist, and he was eventually admitted to a locked treatment facility. When I interviewed him, in order to help him move into a community residence from a locked facility (given the pending closure of the facility), I asked what he needed to be successful in the community. He articulated a list of needs that would help him to succeed. Among that list was his request that all sharp objects, which he would normally use to hurt himself, be removed from his immediate vicinity. He also asked whether tall walls or fences could surround the home so he wouldn't be tempted to run away. Staff members also reported that he was most likely to elope or engage in self-injury whenever he had some kind of strong emotional response. Instead of talking about it, he would act on those feelings. After all, strong emotions can lead to strong impulses. What he was articulating during the interview was clearly the need for a self-care plan to ensure his physical safety when he felt emotionally overwhelmed. He knew he needed to feel safe with himself. He was asking that external controls be introduced in his environment to ensure he did not injure himself. He was able to articulate his needs, but not everyone with an intellectual disability possesses the verbal skills he possessed.

Physical Safety

How many times have individuals with developmental disabilities been admitted to homes with peers who were physically assaultive or who engage in property destruction? Imagine living with individuals who engaged in those behaviors in your own home? Most likely, you would evict them, or move, because the experiences would be too anxiety provoking or stressful. However, there is often a lack of thought or consideration given to promoting a sense of safety when people with developmental disabilities and trauma histories are admitted into group homes or other facilities. Admission is often based on the need for an out-of-home placement, and sometimes there is a need for an emergency placement. However, by doing so, we may be compromising the individual's sense of physical safety, if the individual has a trauma history. If the individual did not have a trauma history upon admission, he or she may experience trauma after admission when confronted with other residents who are exhibiting dangerous or threatening behaviors. When considering admission to an adult residential facility for an individual with a developmental disability (if one is needed and available in the state where the individual resides), it is important to consider the individual's trauma history and whether or not that person is currently exhibiting trauma-based reactions. Otherwise, forcing an individual to reside in an unsafe environment may hinder the individual's ability to heal from their past.

FEELING SAFE WITH OTHERS

What comes to mind when discussing this topic is the concept of boundaries. Boundaries keep us safe in the world. Healthy boundaries are an essential component of mental health and can include emotional, physical, and financial boundaries. Establishing healthy emotional boundaries ensures that people are not being taken advantage of by others, being emotionally abused, or being emotionally injured in some way. Physical boundaries help to maintain a person's physical integrity and guard against physical or sexual abuse. Establishing healthy financial boundaries help people meet their needs for some of the basics in life and more. If financial boundaries are not established, people can overspend. They can lend too much money to others, and they can find themselves operating at a financial deficit and unable to meet their own financial needs. Consequently, it is important for individuals with intellectual disabilities to be supported by individuals who are able to maintain and promote healthy boundaries in all of these arenas. It is also important for the individuals who support them to teach and role model healthy boundaries.

If the individual lives in a residential facility supported by staff, it is important that staff are consistent, reliable, and responsive. It is also important for the same conditions to exist if the individual lives with family or relatives. For individuals with intellectual disabilities and trauma histories to feel safe with people, it is important that they feel listened to and that they feel that their emotional and social needs can be met.

In discussing boundaries, an important concept that is linked to this topic is the concept of responsibility. It is important in supporting individuals with developmental disabilities that boundary training also includes engendering a sense of responsibility for their actions so that they do not always blame others. It involves the use of establishing consequences for specific actions as well as setting limits. As noted by Cloud & Townsend (1995) in their book, *Boundaries*, "Discipline is an external boundary designed to develop internal boundaries in our children. It provides a structure of safety until the child has structure enough in his character to not need it" (p. 140).

Yet, how many times have individuals with developmental disabilities been protected from experiencing the consequences of their actions? This may have been done by well-meaning individuals in the person's life, but consider the long-term consequences of those immediate, well intentioned actions. This author recalls a poignant conversation with a young man who was diagnosed with a mild intellectual disability and a traumatic brain injury. While living in a group home, he would destroy property during some of his anger outbursts. He would often throw items or break them. The administrator for the home simply kept repairing or replacing the items. The individual was not held responsible for either fixing or replacing any of the broken items. Upon leaving the home and moving back to live with his family, he continued these incidents of property destruction when he became very angry. However, this time his parents held him accountable for some of the damages. He broke a door and his father took him to the store to price doors and to assist in replacing the door. A certain percentage of his monthly earnings were given to his parents to assist in fixing the damage he had done. Money was so important to this person that it took only a time or two before incidents of property destruction stopped. He wanted to spend money on the items he enjoyed and on buying presents for his girlfriend. During one of our interviews, he started to tell me how much items would cost to be replaced around the house if he broke them in a fit of anger. He said (pointing to the new indoor window shutters), "That cost a lot of money...like hundreds of dollars. I can't break that." He also said, "Why did they let me do that at the group home? I would have learned not to do that anymore? Why didn't they help me?"

Boundaries help to foster a sense of safety and predictability. By introducing, maintaining, and role modeling healthy boundaries with individuals with intellectual disabilities, care providers help to promote a sense of safety which is a primary need. The individual being supported knows what to expect, and the establishment and maintenance of healthy boundaries by their care providers helps to promote a sense of comfort and protection.

SPECIFIC THERAPIES FOR THE TREATMENT OF PTSD

There are a variety of treatments used to treat posttraumatic stress disorder in the general population. Based on the many research studies published on this topic during the past two decades, there are now evidence-based, trauma-focused interventions available. In 2010, the United States Department of Veterans Affairs, in collaboration with the United States Department of Defense and with the assistance of 56 professional reviewers, identified a list of clinical practice guidelines of psychotherapies which are considered to be the first-line treatments for PTSD (Baranowsky & Gentry, 2014). The therapies included Eye Movement Desensitization and Reprocessing (EMDR), cognitive-based therapies, Stress Inoculation Training (SIT), and exposure-based therapies including prolonged exposure therapy and brief eclectic psychotherapy (Baranowsky & Gentry, 2014). Several of these first-line treatments have also been modified for use with individuals with intellectual disabilities. There have been studies that have been conducted regarding the effectiveness of some of these first-line treatments for use in this population. However, the studies have been sparse and often limited to case studies.

In addition to these front line treatments, there are a variety of other treatment approaches that can be used to address PTSD symptoms and sub-threshold symptoms in the general population. However, the studies on the use of these techniques among individuals with developmental disabilities are also sparse compared to the studies that have been published on their use among the general population (Cooper et al., 2007). There continues to be a lack of systematic studies on the various treatment modalities and the effectiveness of their use with individuals with ID. However, from the limited studies which have been published, including case studies, clinical evidence would suggest that the range of therapeutic approaches that are available to treat PTSD in the general population can also be used with individuals with intellectual disabilities (Focht-New, Clements, Barol, Faulkner, & Pekala, 2008; McCarthy, 2001; Ryan, 1994). However, modifications may need to be made to some of the treatment protocols due to the cognitive limitations associated with intellectual disabilities.

Given the lack of controlled studies regarding the effectiveness of various types of treatments for PTSD among individuals with ID, therapists are often left to extrapolate from the research findings from the general population to this population. They are left to apply some of the same therapeutic approaches used with the general population, make the necessary adaptations to the techniques, and hope for equally promising results. More rigorous, controlled studies are sorely needed not only to establish the effectiveness of each approach but also to compare the various therapeutic approaches. Given the increased prevalence rate of psychiatric disorders among this population and the greater risks for various types of abuse, there is an even greater demand for psychological treatment for individuals with intellectual disabilities. The following sections highlight some of the first-line treatments as well as adjunctive treatments (i.e., supplemental treatments) that are available for use by therapists.

PTSD TREATMENT APPROACHES FOR INDIVIDUALS WITH INTELLECTUAL DISABILITIES

The following therapies, which include eye movement desensitization reprocessing (EMDR), cognitive-behavior therapy, stress inoculation therapy (SIT), and dialectical behavior therapy (DBT), can be used with individuals whose intellectual disabilities are in the mild to moderate range of intellectual functioning and are considered more of the first line treatments. However, there are other adjunctive or supplemental therapies which can also be used for individuals with PTSD and ID such as neurofeedback and yoga. Other therapies that provide a more behavioral, supportive, sensory-based, and somatic approach are more appropriate for individuals whose levels of intellectual functioning lie within the lower ranges of severe and profound intellectual disabilities. These individuals usually lack the language skills to participate in some of the therapies that require verbal skills, as well as the cognitive skills. Consequently, the therapies that include supportive approaches, sensory based, and behavioral interventions are focused more on creating safe environments for the individuals, removing trauma triggers, and providing soothing and relaxing strategies to calm down physical arousal and anxieties.

The following are some of the therapies that can be used for individuals functioning within the mild to moderate range of ID:

Eye Movement Desensitization and Reprocessing (EMDR)

This is a very specific and well researched therapy that is used to treat posttraumatic stress disorder. Eye movement desensitization reprocessing was a therapy developed by Dr. Francine Shapiro in 1987. Its procedures were clinically tested and later published in 1989 in the *Journal of Traumatic Stress*. Since then, its efficacy has been established through numerous studies (Mevissen & de Jongh, 2010; Seidler & Wagner, 2006). She developed it after walking and noticing that her own distressing thoughts decreased after her eyes followed the waves of lines in a fence (Shapiro, 1989). She then argued that lateral eye movements facilitated the reprocessing of traumatic memories which facilitated healing. However, Dr. Shapiro later changed some of her thoughts on the actual necessity of the lateral movements and felt that the changes may have also been the result of other factors which included a cognitive component.

This therapeutic approach was originally called EMD for eye movement desensitization, but in 1991 Dr. Shapiro renamed it eye movement desensitization and reprocessing. This change also reflects the information processing theory that she used to explain its effects. EMDR incorporates an integrative approach, and as Gilderthorp (2015) has noted this approach involves several theoretical approaches including a cognitive component, a behavioral component, and a psychodynamic element. EMDR consists of eight phases:
- Phase 1: History and Treatment Planning
- Phase 2: Preparation
- Phase 3: Assessment
- Phase 4: Desensitization
- Phase 5: Installation
- Phase 6: Body Scan
- Phase 7: Closure
- Phase 8: Reevaluation

After the assessment phase is completed the therapist introduces the use of bilateral stimulation (BLS) which is accomplished by having the person engage in a series of horizontal eye movements which are similar to the rapid eye movements which occur during sleep. However, bilateral stimulation can also occur through the use of auditory or tactile stimuli. While the individual is thinking of a particular memory that is traumatic, the therapist will guide the individual through a set of bilateral stimulation exercises such as a series of eye movements. The client is then asked to rate his or her distress on a scale of 1-10 referred to as Subjective Units of Distress Scale (SUDS). This cycle is repeated until the individual reports a rating of 0 or 1 on the SUD Scale and the person is no longer reporting distress while recalling the memories. This desensitization phase is then followed by an installation phase. After the individual reports very low ratings of distress, he or she is instructed to think of an alternative thought that is positive which is now associated with the imaginal recall of the traumatic event. The client then rates the new positive thought in terms of how much they believe it. The cycle is repeated which includes having the positive thoughts occur using a combination of imagery and bilateral stimulation. This continues until the person endorses a number using a rating scale that suggests a high belief in the new thought (Gilderthorp, 2015; Shapiro, 2001).

There have been numerous studies that have been conducted demonstrating its efficacy for use among the general population (Mevissen & de Jongh, 2010; Seidler & Wagner, 2006). Various organizations have also recognized it as one of the first line treatments for PTSD including the Department of Veterans Affairs, the International Society for the Study of Traumatic Stress, and the American Psychological Association. This treatment modality has also been used to treat PTSD among individuals with intellectual disabilities. The studies investigating its effectiveness for use with this population are sparse in comparison to the number of studies conducted on its efficacy for use in the general population. The studies conducted on its use with individuals with intellectual disabilities are often case studies lacking the more rigorous controlled research methods that have been conducted in the general population. However, the limited studies which have been conducted have yielded promising results, and the standard protocol for the use of EMDR has been modified for use with individuals with intellectual disabilities. Guidelines for modifying its use with individuals with intellectual disabilities have been outlined by the EMDR International Association and include some of the following adaptations:

- Individuals with intellectual disabilities should be allowed to spend more time in the preparation phase.
- When using the Subjective Units of Distress Scale (SUDS), it may be helpful to use a visual representation of the scale. If necessary, the scale can be modified from a scale of 1-10 to a scale numbering 1-5. In addition, pictures of faces showing varying levels of distress can be depicted alongside the various numbers.
- The use of frequent positive reinforcement is recommended in the sessions.
- Role playing and modeling should be used when necessary to reinforce the concepts.

It is interesting to note that Bergmann (2008) proposed that the use of bilateral stimulation resulted in a type of "jump start" of the brain into moving or accessing material that may have been stored in "a mute part of the brain" which does not normally deal with words. Based on this theory, EMDR may be well suited for use in individuals with intellectual disabilities who may have language deficits.

While the published literature on its use among individuals with intellectual disabilities is limited, what has been published has been promising. Mevissen, Lievegoed, and de Jongh (2011) noted that only eight case studies had been published on the use of EMDR with individuals with intellectual disabilities. In response to the dearth of research in the area, Mevissen et al. (2011) conducted an investigation on the applicability of EMDR for the treatment of PTSD with four individuals with mild intellectual disability. The types of trauma that each participant in the study had experienced had varied. Upon completion of the treatment, investigators found a reduction in PTSD symptoms. The treatment gains had maintained at follow-ups which were conducted at 3 months and extended up to 2.5 years. In addition to the reduction in PTSD symptoms, they also reported that the participants in the study had shown improvements in their social and adaptive skills, and a reduction in depressive symptoms, as well as somatic complaints.

In his article on application of EMDR in people with mild intellectual disability, Tharner (2006) reported on the treatment of 20 clients, 10 of whom were diagnosed with PTSD and 9 with complex PTSD (which is condition that is caused by chronic or prolonged exposure to traumatic conditions). Eighty percent of the sample were successfully treated. Successful treatment was defined as the ability of the client to recall the traumatic event without experiencing significant distress or disturbance.

Giltaij (2004) published two case studies. One of the studies involved using EMDR to treat a blind woman with a mild intellectual disability who had been sexually assaulted. The other case involved a 16-year-old girl who had vision deficits and witnessed her sister physically threatening their mother with knives. Giltaij reported that the symptoms of PTSD remitted after four sessions of treatment with EMDR in the first case. When a three month follow-up was conducted, the progress had maintained, and the client was still symptom free. However, with regard to research methods, the investigator did not provide information on how the results were actually measured or how PTSD had been diagnosed. Twelve sessions of EMDR were used with the 16-year-old girl. The young girl then self-reported a decrease in problem severity in several problem areas from a rating of 9 to a 1 (on a self-reporting scale from 1-10).

Gilderthorp (2015) also conducted a review of studies that involved the administration of EMDR for people diagnosed with an intellectual disability. Five studies were evaluated and it was noted that the articles provided "reasons to be optimistic" about the use of this treatment among this population, but the review also stated that more rigorous research is needed.

There was also a case study done by Barrowcliff and Evans (2015) in which an individual with moderate-severe intellectual disability, who was blind and had mucopolysaccharidosis, was treated with EMDR for chronic posttraumatic stress disorder. They implemented the eight phase EMDR interventions, but they modified the techniques because of the individual's cognitive and sensory impairments. The researchers reported a decrease in PTSD symptoms after a series of meetings to prepare the client followed by four session of EMDR.

Barol and Seubert (2010) also conducted an exploratory study of the use of EMDR among six individuals with intellectual disabilities. They used the standard EMDR protocol and made adaptations as needed for each participant.

- **Cognitive Behavioral TherapyCognitive Behavioral Therapy (CBT)**

Cognitive behavior therapy (CBT) is a well-researched treatment approach that has been used to address posttraumatic stress disorder symptoms (Barrowcliff, 2008; Oathamshaw & Haddock, 2006). This form of therapy, which can be done using an individual or group format, proposes that our thoughts and beliefs influence our emotions. Consequently, if we change our thoughts, attitudes, and beliefs, we can influence or change our emotions. • Cognitive Behavioral TherapyCognitive behavioral therapy can be particularly useful for treating anger-related PTSD. Since the anger response has three components consisting of the physical response, cognitions, and behaviors, CBT can be very helpful in identifying the thoughts or cognitions that are contributing to the angry responses. Such cognitions could include inaccurate appraisals of the situation, negative appraisals, or distorted ways of viewing a situation (referred to as "cognitive distortions").

- Cognitive Behavioral TherapyCognitive behavioral therapy is not simply viewing situations from a positive perspective. It challenges the accuracy of someone's thinking, and it can help to identify distorted or inaccurate patterns of thinking. The individual can then focus on replacing those thoughts with more accurate patterns of thinking that can have a positive impact on emotional well-being.

When using this therapeutic approach with individuals with intellectual disability, modifications need to be made in response to the cognitive limitations of the client. Since it focuses on identifying, monitoring, and challenging self-talk (i.e., our internal dialogues), it would not be appropriate for use with individuals whose cognitive functioning abilities lie within the more severe or profound ranges. Barrowcliff (2008) discussed some modifications that can be made to support individuals with lower age equivalents but who are old enough to recognize the connection between thoughts and emotion (Joyce, Globe, & Moody, 2006). Modifications may include helping the individual to discriminate between internal and external dialogue by using visual depictions. For example, using favorite cartoon characters with balloons above their characters depicting thoughts (i.e., thought balloons) may be one method to assist clients with intellectual disabilities in identifying internal dialogues.

There have been a few studies published on the use of cognitive behavior therapy (CBT) among individuals with ID within the mild range of cognitive functioning with some evidence that it can be effective for reducing symptoms across a number of psychiatric conditions including anxiety and depression (Lemmon & Mizes, 2002; Pert, Jahoda, & Stenfert, 2013; Unwin, Tsimopoulou, Stenfert, & Asmi, 2016). However, fewer have been published on its use in addressing PTSD in this population. Among the general population, studies have found it to be effective in reducing PTSD symptoms. However, some researchers have found that it is not as effective with individuals who have suffered multiple or prolonged traumatic experiences and who have poor verbal memories (Carr, 2011).

Stress Inoculation Therapy (SIT)

This is a form of • Cognitive Behavioral Therapycognitive behavioral therapy that was developed by Meichenbaum (1975). It has also been referred to as stress exposure training. It has multiple components and a broad range of use. It has been used to treat trauma and lessen PTSD symptoms, as well as to treat anger management issues, stress, and anxiety. There are many studies that have examined its use and effectiveness with individuals suffering from PTSD in the general population (Veronen & Kilpatrick, 1982). It has also been used with individuals with intellectual disability to address aggression and issues with controlling angry impulses. Malcolm & Hiebert (1986) published a case study of its use in decreasing the anger outbursts of a 30-year-old individual with an intellectual disability. Tantrum behavior decreased at the end of the treatment.

It has been used both as a treatment approach as well as a preventative approach. With PTSD, it has also been used as an adjunct or supplemental treatment to other interventions to treat the disorder. A central principle underlying the use of SIT is the concept of inoculation which has also been used in medicine. As with the concept of vaccinations in the medical field, this therapy is based on the premise that if an individual is gradually exposed to milder forms of the stressful situations it can provide an opportunity to improve coping skills. By preparing ahead of time with the identification of strategies that can be used to cope with PTSD symptoms and stressful situations, the person is, in essence, inoculating him or herself again future stressors.

Stress inoculation therapy consists of three stages which include the educational phase, the skill acquisition state, and finally, its application period. During the first phase, the person is educated on the approach and the rationale for its use. During the second phase, specific coping skills are identified which the individual can practice. It is an individually tailored intervention driven by the type of stressors the individual has encountered. With the therapist, the client identifies possible high risk stressful situations they may encounter. The therapist helps the individual to become aware of specific triggers that can trigger trauma-related fears, anxieties, or stress reactions. A variety of coping skills are identified which the individual can use when confronted with the stressful situations. Inevitably, the coping skills would include some form of relaxation training exercises in order to calm down the individual's physical arousal which can accompany stress or anxiety. Such techniques may then include breathing techniques for relaxation, identifying and changing self-talk or thoughts, the use of imagery, behavioral rehearsal, guided self-dialogue, cue controlled relaxation, role-modeling, and problem-solving. Assertiveness training skills are sometimes also incorporated into the strategies depending upon the needs of the client. The coping strategies that are identified are individually determined. The coping skills can be practiced and role-played before the cues for the trauma-related fears are encountered. During the final phase, the person will use the coping strategies in the high risk situations.

Dialectical Behavior Therapy (DBT)

Dialectical Behavior Therapy is a therapeutic approach originally developed by Dr. Marsha Linehan (1993) to treat individuals diagnosed with borderline personality disorder. It is a modification of • Cognitive Behavioral Therapycognitive behavioral therapy. It incorporates aspects of behavioral therapy, dialectical philosophy, and practices derived from Buddhism (Lynch, Trost, Salsmann, & Linehan, 2007).

People who have been diagnosed with this personality disorder experience a great deal of instability in their relationships, mood, and behavior. The personality disorder is characterized by emotional dysregulation, interpersonal conflicts, and behavioral and cognitive dysregulation. Dialectical behavior therapy was designed to help develop regulation skills in these areas. Since its development, its use has expanded to treat different types of psychiatric disorders, in addition to borderline personality disorder, including treating individuals with various mood disorders, addictive disorders, traumatic brain injuries, as well as PTSD.

The skills training approach of DBT is geared towards improving emotional regulation and decreasing any self-destructive behaviors. This treatment approach helps to decrease the symptoms of PTSD among individuals in the general population. It teaches people to help manage their emotions through a variety of skills and to decrease any unhealthy coping methods. DBT theory suggests that there are people whose level of emotional arousal can increase faster than the average person and remain at elevated levels for longer periods of time.

Dialectical behavior therapy has four main components: mindfulness, distress tolerance training, emotional regulation training, and interpersonal effectiveness training. This approach is skill based, and it uses a combination of weekly individual therapy sessions as well as group sessions. According to Merra (2005), "DBT presumes that the intensity of affect is caused by dialectical conflict between self and environment defined as inadequate compromises between competing needs and wants, attachment, trauma and loss experience of the patient or genetic kindling effects" (p. 6).

There have been modifications or adaptations of the DBT interventions for individuals with developmental disabilities. For example, Dykstra and Charlton (2003) proposed modifications in an unpublished manuscript entitled, *Dialectical Behavior Therapy Skills Training: Adapted for Special Populations*. Their adaptations focused primarily on children with developmental disabilities in their piloted study. However, the modifications they have proposed have also been recommended and used by other researchers not only for children with developmental disabilities but also with adults (Hurley, Tomasulo, & Pfadt, 1998; Lew, Matta, Tripp-Tebo, & Watts, 2006). The modifications that have been made for use with individuals with intellectual disabilities still contain the same tenets of DBT, but the trainings have been adapted to facilitate comprehension. The language has been modified and the skills training components simplified for ease of understanding, and the training includes more repetition, feedback, and rehearsal.

Mindfulness

Mindfulness is a concept found in some of the Eastern philosophies such as Buddhism. It refers to the process by which one is focused on what is occurring in the moment. Mindfulness training involves teaching people to fully experience what is occurring in the present. It involves maintaining a moment-by-moment awareness of thoughts, feelings, and physical responses or sensations when involved in an activity or task and doing so in a non-judgmental manner (Kabat-Zinn, Massion, Kristeller, & Peterson, 1992). Whatever someone is doing at that moment should have his or her full awareness. For example, if someone were washing the car and practicing mindfulness, he or she would concentrate on how the water and soap felt as the car was being washed and other aspects of the task. The individual would be concentrating only on the task at hand and not be thinking about what other tasks need to be done that day or thinking about something totally unrelated. Washing the car would occupy the person's full senses.

Mindfulness has been incorporated into several different therapeutic interventions including dialectical behavior therapy. Studies have shown the effectiveness of practicing mindfulness in helping to alleviate symptoms of PTSD as well as alleviating symptoms of depression and anxiety (Kabat-Zinn et al., 1992; Segal, Williams, & Teasdale, 2002). It strengthens emotional regulation, and it can reduce stress. This is a very useful technique not only to help treat a variety of psychiatric conditions but as a strategy for daily use, in general. It is an intervention that has been used in the general population as well as with individuals with intellectual disabilities. Mindfulness-based interventions with modifications have been used with individuals whose cognitive functioning abilities have ranged from the mild to profound levels. Among individuals with intellectual disabilities it has also been used to address a variety of behavioral challenges including aggression and self-injury. Singh et al. (2007) used mindfulness training to assist individuals with intellectual disabilities in the moderate range using a mindfulness procedure called "meditations on the soles of the feet" with three individuals whose level of ID was in the moderate range. They were at risk of losing their community placements due to aggressive behavior. The intervention proved effective with modifications to the protocol, and the individuals were able to maintain their placements. During this exercise the individual was instructed to stand, sit, or walk slowly and to start thinking about the incident that got them mad. While thinking about it, the participant was then instructed to shift attention to the soles of their feet paying careful attention to details of this experience such as feeling the texture of the socks, the feel of the shoes, the feel of the floor, etc. The individual was instructed to breathe normally and keep the focus until calm. Although usually used for individuals with mild ID, Singh et al. (2007) modified this for use with individuals with moderate ID because they were having more difficulty moving beyond the anger.

Although mindfulness is now being embraced as an additional treatment for PTSD among the general population, there is a lack of empirical studies regarding its use with individuals with intellectual disability. However, it may hold promise since it helps individuals to focus on what is occurring in the present and not on the trauma that has occurred in the past. Further research would be needed to assess its true efficacy in alleviating PTSD symptoms or trauma-related stress symptoms among this population.

Meditation

Meditation can be used to help improve emotional regulation and as a complementary therapy for the treatment of PTSD alongside other treatments. It activates the parasympathetic nervous system which is the part of the nervous system that calms down arousal. Research shows that when meditating there is an increase in theta waves which is the type of brain activity associated with calmness (Lutz, Greischar, Rawlings, Ricard, & Davidson, 2004).

There are different types of meditation. Transcendental Meditation (TM) is one form of meditation which has been the subject of a substantial body of research studies documenting its health and emotional benefits. It has been shown to reduce blood pressure (Barnes, Schneider, Alexander, & Staggers, 1997), to reduce cardiac mortality, stress, anxiety (Alexander et al., 1993; Eppley & Abrams, 1989), and to reduce symptoms of PTSD among war veterans (Barnes, Rigg, & Williams, 2013; Rosenthal, Grosswald, Ross, & Rosenthal, 2011).

There continues to be a lack of controlled studies on its use in reducing PTSD symptoms and traumatic stress responses in individuals with intellectual disabilities. However, there have been a few case studies published which have noted its positive impact among this population in terms of reducing a variety of symptoms. Eyerman (1981) published a case study discussing its positive impact on a 26-year-old female who was diagnosed with an intellectual disability in the moderate range. After practicing TM over the course of three years, improvements were noted in her social behavior as well as in her verbal skills and health. In a more recent study of its effects when used with individuals with autism spectrum disorder (ASD), Black & Rosenthal (2015) presented six case studies conducted with children and adults ranging in ages from 10 to 30 who had been diagnosed with ASD. The participants practiced Transcendental Meditation twice daily for approximately 15-20 minutes during each session. The participants found it easy to learn and use consistently. It is a simple form of meditation that requires no adherence to a specific philosophy. The individuals discussed in the case studies reported a variety of benefits including improved concentration, improved sleep, a reduction in anxiety, and a reduction in physical symptoms of stress.

Although there is a lack of systematic and case studies regarding the use of meditation among individuals with ID, who have either PTSD or subthreshold symptoms of PTSD, it may hold some promise for improving emotional regulation and decreasing some of the physiological signs and symptoms of stress. It may be a viable treatment option for individuals who have mild to moderate intellectual disabilities.

Psychodynamic Psychotherapy

This approach has also been referred to as insight oriented therapy. It examines such factors as the influence that the past can have on present behaviors. It examines unresolved conflicts, and it focuses on different factors that can contribute to, or influence, PTSD symptoms. For example, it may focus on childhood relationships and experiences and the conflicts in current relationships and how such experiences may be impacting PTSD symptoms (Schottenbauer, Glass, Arnkoff, & Gray, 2008). There is no specific protocol for this type of treatment. To date, there are only a small number of case studies published that suggest its usefulness with some individuals with trauma history. For example, Razza (1997) discussed its use in treating PTSD symptoms with a woman who had been diagnosed with a mild intellectual disability and a history of sexual abuse in childhood. Case studies have reported some positive results for use with individuals with intellectual disabilities and trauma histories (Cottis, 2008).

Neurofeedback

Neurofeedback, also referred to as EEG biofeedback, has been in use since 1960. It was first used to treat PTSD in the 1980's, but it has also been used to treat a variety of conditions including physical conditions such as migraines and psychiatric conditions such as attention deficit disorder and anxiety disorders. With neurofeedback an individual is trained to teach his or her brain to regulate stress by turning off the stress response and changing brain waves. It provides a guided form of feedback in which the individual learns to control brain ways via a brain-computer interface. By receiving information or feedback about changes in one's brain's electrical activity, an individual can learn to change brain waves to induce a more calm state.

Studies have shown some effectiveness after a series of neurofeedback sessions in decreasing symptoms of PTSD as an alternative method of treatment. A study by van der Kolk et al. (2016) indicated that when compared to a control group of individuals who did not receive the treatment, individuals who did undergo sessions of neurofeedback showed a significant decrease in PTSD symptoms. Participants in the study also showed improvements in their abilities to regulate their emotions.

There have numerous studies conducted on the use of neurofeedback in the treatment of ADHD, but its success in addressing other neurodevelopmental disorders is not as well studied (Duric, Assmus, Gundersen, & Elgen, 2012; Meisel, Servera, Garcia-Banda, Cardo, & Moreno, 2013). There are only a handful of studies that have researched its impact on individuals with intellectual disabilities and a lack of studies specifically focusing on its use in decreasing PTSD symptoms in individuals with intellectual disabilities. For example, Hong and Lee (2012) investigated the effects of neurofeedback training on attentional processes among 21 children who were diagnosed with intellectual abilities. The participants were assigned to one of three groups consisting of a neurofeedback training group, a no treatment or control group, and a visual perception training group. The neurofeedback training group showed significant improvement in all test scores, and neurofeedback training was found to be an effective way to improve attention among the participants. Surmeli and Ertem (2007) used neurofeedback training to help eight children (ages 6-14) who were diagnosed with Down syndrome. The purpose of their study was to see if neurofeedback training would be helpful in improving attention, memory, speech, and language and in decreasing impulsivity and behavioral challenges. One participant dropped out of the study, and the remaining seven children completed the neurofeedback training and showed statistically significant improved in all of the identified areas.

Yoga

Yoga has been used as an adjunct treatment for a variety of psychiatric disorders including posttraumatic stress disorder. Yoga is an ancient practice that is thought to have emerged from India. It involves training the mind and body to achieve a better balance. It includes the use of various breathing exercises, physical postures, and meditation. Various postures are used to improve concentration, increase blood flow to the brain, and improve flexibility. It has been used to treat a variety of both psychological and physical disorders, and it has been used as an integrative approach and an adjunctive approach to treating PTSD. The International Association of Yoga Therapists (IAYT) has published guidelines for the training of yoga therapists (Libby, Reddy, Pilver, & Desai, 2012).

Yoga can be used as a complement to other therapies that are being used to address PTSD symptoms among the general population as well as among individuals with intellectual disabilities. Yoga is being used in several Veterans Administrations programs, and its impact on the symptoms of PTSD has undergone numerous studies. Yoga is becoming increasingly recognized as an effective treatment for reducing PTSD symptoms (Miller, 2009; Pollack, 2010; van der Kolk, 2006).

Although there is an expanding awareness of the effectiveness of using yoga as an adjunct treatment among the general population, there are only a few studies examining its effectiveness when used among individuals with developmental disabilities. According to the studies which have been published, the results are promising, but they have not been extended to include controlled studies on its impact on PTSD symptoms. For example, there was a study conducted in India in by Uma, Nagendra, Nagarathna, Vaidehi, & Seethalakshmi (1989). It was a one year controlled study. Ninety children with varying degrees of intellectual disabilities including mild, moderate, and severe levels participated in the study from four special schools located in Bangalore, India. Of those children, 45 underwent yoga training for one academic year. They participated for five hours every week with an integrated set of yoga practices including breathing exercises. The study included a control group of forty-five other children who were matched for chronological age, sex, IQ, socioeconomic status, and socio environment background. Individuals in the control group were not exposed to yoga training but continued in their usual school routine for the period of one year. At the end of the study, the yoga group showed significant improvements in social adaptation parameters being measured in the study as well as improved IQ scores as compared to the control group.

There are different forms of yoga and some individuals with intellectual disabilities and physical limitations may not be able to practice all of the poses. Some of the poses may need to be modified. Several different types of yoga which have been used have included Hatha Yoga and Yoga Nidra (a form of deep relaxation).

Relaxation Response Training

Relaxation skills training can involve several different strategies. As a way to facilitate relaxation and decrease levels of emotional arousal, there have been numerous studies documenting the benefits of diaphragmatic breathing exercises (Lee et al., 2003). Diaphragmatic breathing, otherwise known as deep breathing or belly breathing, is a breathing technique which is done by contracting the diaphragm. When performing this breathing exercise, an individual is instructed to breathe slowly and deeply through the nose allowing the abdomen to rise and the chest to rise. It is important that the abdomen rises with inhalation. Exhalation is done slowly through the mouth. It is sometimes helpful to instruct the individual to place his or her hand on the stomach so that upon inhale the stomach moves out against the hand. Upon exhale the individual is instructed to pull in their abdomen. The individual can perform this exercise while either lying down or sitting comfortably (while maintaining a good posture). It can also be done while standing. Sometimes it is helpful to practice this breathing exercise with eyes closed for increased awareness. Belly breathing strengthens the diaphragm and encourages a full oxygen exchange. The individual can practice by taking 10 seconds for the inhalation followed by a brief pause and then 10 seconds for the exhalation. This trial is then repeated several times for at least 5-10 minutes for each session. This should be practiced several times a day. If it becomes part of a daily routine, it is more likely to be practiced. The instructions can also be recorded. Establishing it as a daily routine can be particularly helpful for individuals with intellectual disabilities because of the deficits in executive functioning that occurs with intellectual disabilities. These deficits can result in difficulties with planning and initiating tasks.

Exposure Therapy

Exposure therapy began as a form of therapy in the 1980's, and it has been used to treat individuals who suffer from PTSD. With PTSD, individuals may develop fears of being in certain environments because they are concerned that memories of the trauma may return. Consequently, they may avoid specific environments because the reminders may trigger distress. Exposure therapy is used to reintroduce them to the feared situations or the situations they have been avoiding.

There are two types of exposure therapy. One form is referred to as flooding. This involves a rapid exposure to the feared situations. Using this approach, the individual is exposed to the anxiety-producing stimuli with the belief that with enough exposure to the feared situation, the anxiety would lessen. Flooding may result in exposing the individual to the feared situation for as long as several hours. The second approach to exposure therapy involves a graduated exposure to the feared situations which is known as systematic desensitization or a progressive exposure. The goal of systematic desensitization is to help the individual lessen the fears and avoidance behaviors. This is done by gradually exposing the individual to the environment in such progressive increments that he or she is not overwhelmed by the experience. This allows the individual more control over the length and the frequency of the exposures to the anxiety-provoking situations.

Systematic desensitization consists of several main elements which include relaxation training and the development of a desensitization hierarchy. When constructing a desensitization hierarchy, the individual creates a fear hierarchy which is a list that begins with the least feared aspects of the situation and progresses to the most anxiety provoking aspects of the situation (which is avoided due to trauma). Exposure treatments are paired with different relaxation techniques so as to lessen or remove the anxiety.

Exposure therapy can be done through an in vivo exposure (i.e., in real life) or by imaginal exposure in which the individual imagines being exposed to the feared situation. If accomplished through an in vivo procedure, the individual would face the feared environment in real life. For example, if someone was assaulted in a particular part of the city and responded by avoiding that area, the use of an in vivo exposure procedure (using a systematic desensitization approach) would have the person gradually return to that specific area. If exposure therapy is done through imaginal desensitization, an individual develops a hierarchy of steps in their imagination that gradually exposes him or her to the environments that had been avoided. This can be followed by in vivo exposure in which the individual actually encounters those environments in real life. Systematic desensitization has been used to treat not only PTSD or traumatic responses involving avoidance but also a variety of phobias.

For individuals whose cognitive functioning levels are within the lower ranges of intellectual disabilities, such as in the profound and severe range, imaginal desensitization would be inappropriate. However, a behavioral approach may be used whereby a therapist can gradually try to expose the individual to the feared situations by pairing the feared stimulus with positive experiences, thereby changing the conditioning associated with the fear or anxiety. For individuals whose cognitive functioning abilities lie within the mild to moderate range, imaginal as well as in vivo exercises can be done.

When using exposure therapy, it is important that the therapist proceed slowly and cautiously so as to not overwhelm the individual with anxiety and to not overwhelm the individual's ability to cope and manage any emotions which may arise. Consequently, not everyone may be a candidate for this therapy. This therapy was also developed before the advances in neuroscience that discussed the dysregulation that can occur in the nervous system leading to over reactivity and heightened arousal.

As with the other forms of therapy to treat PTSD, there is a paucity of systematic and controlled research on its use among individuals with intellectual disabilities. Lemmon and Mizes (2002) published a study on the use of exposure therapy with an individual with a mild intellectual disability and PTSD who had been sexually assaulted several times. After twenty-five sessions, which were augmented by asking the client to do some homework, the researchers reported she was no longer experiencing distress when she was confronted with trauma-related cues. There was a significant decrease in her anger outbursts and in her hypervigilance.

Sensory Modulation Strategies

Sensory interventions are becoming more widely used in the treatment of trauma as well as in the treatment of other psychiatric disorders (Champagne, 2003). Researchers and practitioners are now moving towards integrating sensory interventions with trauma informed interventions (LeBel, Champagne, Stromberg, & Coyle, 2010). Trauma-informed care is now a model that supports sensory-based practices (Wimer, 2017). This is particularly relevant in addressing PTSD symptoms since this disorder can compromise neurological functioning and produce neural changes in the brain (increased limbic system functioning, decreased frontal lobe functioning, reduced hippocampus, etc.). Because trauma can cause changes in the nervous system, incoming stimuli may be misinterpreted or incorrectly processed. This could lead to an individual overreacting to various situations. It can also produce an under responsiveness to the stimulus. Studies have shown that atypical sensory modulation issues in the form of under- or over-responsiveness, or sensory seeking, may lead to psychological distress (Bar-Shalita & Cermak, 2016). Sensory modulation is the process that follows after the sensory information is registered, interpreted, and integrated by the brain (Kinnealey, Koenig, & Smith, 2011).

Sensory information is received by the nervous system through the five general senses of sight, touch, hearing, taste, and smell, as well as several others. Information is also processed through proprioceptive, vestibular, and interoceptive channels (Wimer, 2017). Proprioception is the ability to sense the body's position in space. It utilizes the compression and traction of joints and muscles. The vestibular system provides us with a sense of balance and equilibrium. Interception involves the sensations that occur in the body such as hunger, pain, thirst, sleepiness, etc.

Given all of these senses, the nervous system needs a certain amount of sensory input referred to as the neurological threshold (Brown & Dunn, 2002). If someone has a high neurological threshold, they are under-responsive to stimuli. Consequently, the individual may require intense sensory stimuli in order to maintain an appropriate threshold. If someone has a low neurological threshold, they tend to be over-responsive, and the person's nervous system can become easily overwhelmed (Brown et al., 2002). According to Kinnealey et al. (2011), dysfunction within this cycle can lead to individuals feeling overwhelmed, disorganized, and irritable if they are overresponsive to stimuli. Some individuals experiencing sensory defensiveness may tend to isolate more and have more symptoms of depression and anxiety.

The use of the sensory modulation model has numerous implications for treating trauma as well as for treating other psychiatric disorders. The identification of underlying sensory issues can be important in understanding someone's behavior. The sensory processing cycle consists of integrating sensory information, followed by sensory discrimination, followed by sensory modulation, and sensory modulation then leads to a behavioral response (Wimer, 2017). Consequently, if there are difficulties in any of the aspects of the cycle, these difficulties can impact behavior.

Sensory techniques and strategies are being used to assist individuals in regulating their emotions and decreasing physiological arousal. Given that posttraumatic stress disorder can result in an overreaction by the nervous system, it is important to consider interventions that can improve emotional self-regulation. This is even more important when supporting individuals with intellectual abilities, given that some of the deficits in executive functioning, which can occur with the disability itself, can produce emotional regulation difficulties. These difficulties can then be compounded by the emotional regulation difficulties that can occur in PTSD. In addition, some individuals with developmental disabilities who have co-existing autism, may have sensory regulation issues as a result of the autism spectrum disorder. Imagine the combined effect of trying to regulate an emotional response if you are an individual with an intellectual disability, who also has autism, and who also has PTSD. It is in situations like this that the importance and benefits of using a multi-disciplinary approach to treating PTSD becomes readily apparent. By accessing the consultation services of an occupational therapist, sensory-based assessment tools can be used to help create a sensory profile for the individual. A sensory profile would help to identify sensory sensitivities, sensory thresholds, etc., so that various sensory modalities and interventions can be identified that can help individual to self-soothe and decrease physiological arousal (Brown & Dunn, 2002).

The use of such sensory-based approaches to help regulate emotions and stabilize behaviors can also form the basis for safety plans for individuals with PTSD or stress-related behaviors, if behavioral challenges begin to escalate. Such sensory interventions could include creating multi-sensory rooms or relaxation rooms, creating a sensory garden, and even the use of weighted modalities such as weighted blankets, weighted vests, weighted stuffed animals, etc. It is interesting to note that studies are now being done on the use of such sensory interventions in psychiatric facilities. For example, Novak, Scanlan, McCaul, MacDonald, and Clarke (2012) created a sensory room on an inpatient psychiatric unit in Australia in an effort to see if it would lower self-reported ratings of distress among the patients and decrease behavioral disturbances. The patients were asked to rate their levels of distress on a scale of 1-10 prior to using the sensory room and after using the room. Other variables were also included in the study such as the use of psychotropic medications, restraint use, duration of the use of the room, and the type of equipment used. The researchers also had the staff rate eleven common behavioral disturbances exhibited by each patient both pre and post room use. In general, the patients reported a mean 2.3 reduction in their self-ratings of distress after using the room with the average duration of room use being 39 minutes. Staff ratings of clients' behavioral disturbances also reflected decreases. Given the high prevalence of trauma among the users of inpatient psychiatric facilities, using such a sensory-based approached is certainly a less invasive and more trauma informed intervention.

Emotional Regulation Skills Training

Emotional self-regulation can be considered as the ability to respond to and manage one's emotions, as well as the behaviors or impulses that can accompany them. It is not an isolated skill but a multifaceted one. With emotional regulation skills, individuals are able to self-soothe and calm themselves down when distressed which is an extremely important skill to possess in today's society. Individuals who are able to regulate the intensity of their emotions are more likely to produce productive and more socially appropriate responses.

Self-regulation skills generally develop over time and are developmental in nature.

When infants are soothed by their parents by either touch or the sound of a reassuring voice, this aids in helping the baby to calm down. Such comforting strategies introduced by the parent help to ensure that the child's nervous system does not remain at a heightened level of arousal. Infants rely on adults to help regulate their emotional responses (Sroufe, 1979). Young children start to learn to inhibit some of the urges which accompany strong emotions in response to what adults teach them to do. For example, a child may be taught to wait his or her turn when playing a game even though they may want to go next. Prompting the child to wait is a way of teaching the child to inhibit impulses and regulate emotional tension (Blair & Diamond, 2008). In addition, when adults have developmentally appropriate expectations for children's behaviors, the children begin to learn to internalize the self-regulating skills. Children also learn emotional regulation skills by watching how adults manage their emotions. As language develops, it also becomes important in helping to regulate emotions. Individuals can talk to themselves and talk to others about a situation. For children who do not have an intellectual disability, language development becomes an important intrinsic method to help regulate emotions (Cole, Michel, & Teti, 1994). As children become older, they also learn more emotional regulation skills as they interact with peers. If they are too emotional and overreactive, they may be rejected by peers. More appropriate and modulated emotional reactions facilitate good peer relationships (Fabes, Einsenberg, Karbon, Troyer, & Switzer, 1994).

Deficits in emotional regulation skills underlie several different psychiatric disorders. Emotional dysregulation is found among individuals diagnosed with borderline personality disorder, various mood disorders, and in trauma-related disorders such as PTSD. Emotional dysregulation can also be found among individuals who have deficits in their executive functioning abilities such as individuals with traumatic brain injuries and individuals with developmental disabilities. Although there are limited studies on emotional regulation skills among individuals with intellectual disabilities, there is some evidence to suggest that individuals with ID lack a repertoire of adequate coping skills when confronted with strong emotions (Benson & Fuchs, 1999). Behavior intervention plans that commonly include the use of contingency management or rewards for certain behaviors do not foster the development of emotional regulation skills. Behavior becomes dependent upon external controls, and the skills do not become intrinsic.

Although more research is needed in this area for individuals with intellectual disabilities, several strategies that can be taken from some of the other therapeutic approaches can be used as part of the training for the developmental of these skills. Developing emotional regulation skills is different than involving coping skills. However, coping does involve regulating emotions. Coping skills are promoted in response to negative events and involve more than affect. Whereas, emotional regulation skills training involves changing affect and directing emotions so that they can be managed in more productive and adaptive ways. Emotional regulation skills can be promoted and taught in various ways such as:
- Care providers (e.g., staff, parents, etc.) can model correct behavior.
- Relaxation strategies can be taught and role modeled.
- Strategies that can improve executive functioning skills such as the development of problem-solving skills can be used to help individuals think through

situations.
- Another strategy that is associated with self-regulation is self-instruction (i.e., self-talk). A person can be taught and encouraged to use self-instruction to help control his or her behavior.
- Board games can also be used to help teach the person to wait and take turns. Such activities can be incorporated into their recreational activities and can also help to build executive functioning skills.
- If the person is functioning within the mild to moderate range of intellectual disabilities, help him or her to identify personal goals and to break them down into small increments which can be achieved. This can help to build executive functioning skills which will also help to build emotional regulation skills. Planning, sequencing, and organizing are all executive, pre-frontal lobe functions. Developing personal goals can even include identifying goals for the day and not just more long-term planning. For example, if a personal goal for the day is to talk to staff when a problem arises, this would help the individual to self-monitor their own behaviors and thoughts. There skills are important to improving one's ability to self-regulate emotions.
- Anger management strategies that include self-monitoring can also be taught. Self-monitoring can include self-observation and then self-reinforcement. For example, if an individual with a mild intellectual disability has intensive outbursts when feeling angry, teaching the individual to self-monitor can be helpful. He or she can be taught to identify levels of anger on a scale of 1-10 with different ratings resulting in different courses of action. For example, if the person feels angry and their self-reported level of anger is at an 8, he or she may want to take a time-out and engage in a distracting activity until the self-reported level drops to a 1 or 2 at which time they may want to talk it out and problem-solve. It would not be beneficial to talk and try to solve the issue when the anger level is reported to be at such a high rating.
- Meditation and mindfulness exercises can also be taught.
- Sensory interventions can be introduced and may be particularly effective for individuals who are non-verbal and cannot articulate how they are feeling.
- Participating in sports can improve both emotional regulation skills and several executive functioning skills. Sports activities can provide opportunities for an individual to learn how to take turns, lose gracefully, and monitor their own actions.
- For individuals with intellectual disabilities in the severe and profound ranges, the use of alternative interventions to language based interventions may be helpful. This could include music therapy, animal assisted therapy, etc., or more sensory based interventions which are approaches that can be helpful in regulating emotional responses.

As Chapman, Shedlack, and France (2006) noted, the de-institutionalization movement has highlighted the need to help individuals with intellectual disabilities develop the self-regulation skills required to successfully integrate into the community. With the closing of many of the institutions, it becomes even more important that individuals with intellectual disabilities learn the skills to control their emotions. This will assist them to not become aggressive or self-destructive and enable them to successfully live with greater freedoms.

Animal Assisted Therapy

The use of animals for therapeutic reasons is not new. The first reported use of animals was noted to have occurred in the late 18th century when they were introduced to patients who were institutionalized (Serpell, 2010). Animal assisted therapy, also known as animal assisted intervention, is one of the therapies now being used to support individuals suffering from trauma or posttraumatic stress disorder. Although dogs are the most common animal use for this form of therapy, other animals such as cats, horses, and birds have also been included. There is now a growing field of equine assisted psychotherapy.

Under the umbrella of animal assisted therapy are other activities such as animal assisted activities. This includes informal interactions between animal handlers and visitors. No treatment goals are identified for these types of interactions. Examples of animal assisted activities may include having animals visit nursing home residents or provide comfort for victims of trauma. However, safety measures and precautions need to still be in place for these types of visits. For example, the handlers need to consider whether the people have any allergies. In addition, the animals' care takers need to ensure that animals are in good health and have a good disposition for such visits. These interactions need to be supervised at all times for the safety of the individuals as well as for the safety of the animals.

Animal assisted therapy is still a burgeoning field and guidelines are still being established and more empirical studies are needed. However, the results of some of the published studies have been encouraging. In fact, the results of animal assisted intervention have been so encouraging in terms of lessening the symptoms of trauma and PTSD that the Department of Defense has been conducting more studies for its use among war veterans. There is also research on the use of this intervention among individuals who are depressed with studies finding it can reduce depressive symptoms (Souter & Miller, 2007).

Studies have shown that when animals are present they tend to facilitate social interaction which can help decrease the sense of loneliness experienced by people with PTSD or trauma (Wood, Giles-Corti, & Bulsara, 2005). Because PTSD can lead to hyperarousal, some studies have shown that the presence of an animal has been linked with an increase in oxytocin in people (Beetz, Uvnas-Moberg, Julius, & Kotrschal, 2012) which can reduce arousal symptoms. O'Haire, Guerin, and Kirkham (2015) conducted a systematic review of the literature on the use of animal assisted intervention. From their review they found that one of the most commonly reported positive outcomes was a reduction in symptoms of depression in 6 out of 10 studies. The second most commonly reported outcome was a decrease in symptoms of PTSD in 5 out of 10 studies. They also found that symptoms of anxiety were reduced with the use of animal assisted intervention. There have also been several studies conducted on the use of animal assisted intervention and its impact on sleep. Newton (2014) found that having the presence of a companion or service dog reduced the frequency of nightmares experienced by veterans, and Nevins, Finch, Hickling, and Barnett (2013) found in their study that the duration of sleep increased with the introduction of animal assisted intervention. A study by Kemp, Signal, Bostros, Taylor, and Prentice (2014) noted a significant reduction of 63% in challenging behaviors among their participant sample of 30 children and adolescents when animals were introduced. A review by O'Haire et al. (2015) indicated that the research to date is largely finding positive results from the use of animal assisted interventions. However, further systematic research with strict methodology is needed to better understand its use and to develop evidence-based animal assisted intervention treatment protocols. In particular, there is a lack of empirical research regarding the use of animal assisted interventions with individuals with intellectual disability suffering from trauma or from PTSD. However, there is some research noting its positive impact on increasing social interaction among children on the autism spectrum (O'Haire, 2013).

It is important to note that there are some limitations and cautions to be considered when using this type of intervention. It can be stressful on the animals. Therefore, the animal handlers need to be attuned to the animal and its reactions in order to avoid causing the animal any unnecessary stress (Serpell, Coppinger, & Fine, 2000). Handlers also need to take into consideration the animal's behavioral needs, physical requirements, and developmental milestones in order to ensure that the interaction with people remains therapeutic. Also, when working with children, children need to be taught how to properly interact with the animals and handle them.

Assertiveness Training Skills

Although this training is not typically referenced in the literature on PTSD among individuals with intellectual disability, it is this author's clinical experience that for some individuals with trauma histories this is an important skill to learn. Assertiveness training allows individuals to build interpersonal skills which can be very empowering for them. The components of assertiveness training include learning the difference between aggressive, assertive, and passive responses. Learning about body language (e.g., threatening versus non-threatening body postures), voice quality, latency, and duration of responses (e.g., impulsive versus more appropriate social responses) can also be part of the instructional training.

Given the vulnerabilities of this population and the high risks for exploitation and abuse, learning assertiveness skills can help to serve as a protection against further incidents of abuse. Assertiveness training has also been shown to reduce stress and improve self-esteem which can facilitate resiliency following traumatic events. It has also been this author's clinical experience that training in this area, coupled with problem-solving skill training, can be an effective intervention for not only decreasing interpersonal conflicts, but decreasing anger outbursts. It can assist the individual in more effectively expressing their wants and needs and ensuring their needs are met.

Nezu, Nezu, and Arean (1991) conducted a study on the effect of assertiveness training with individuals with mild intellectual disabilities who were also dually diagnosed with psychiatric disorders. As a result of the training, participants in the study showed improvements in adaptive functioning, decreased self-reports of distress, and a decrease in anger as well as psychiatric symptoms. As noted by Menolascino (1977) and Reiss and Trenn (1984), individuals with intellectual disabilities often have limited ways of managing interpersonal conflict which can lead to more negative social stress, anxiety, and frustration.

Although there is a lack of controlled studies on the impact of assertiveness training on the symptoms of PTSD or subthreshold PTSD, the tenets of the training are well aligned with the Principles of trauma-informed careprinciples of trauma-informed care. For example, collaboration and mutuality, empowerment and choice, trustworthiness, and safety are all principles of a trauma-informed approach. As individuals learn how to be more assertive, there is a greater likelihood that respect and mutuality can occur in interpersonal interactions. This also helps to build trust.

Music Therapy

Music therapy is one of the expressive therapies, and it is evidence-based. It is the clinical use of interventions to accomplish specific goals for an individual, and it is performed by a credentialed professional. An assessment is done which identifies the individual's strengths and their needs, and a treatment plan is devised.

Music therapy has been used to treat PTSD symptoms. For example, in a small pilot study conducted between 2010 and 2011 by the Veterans Administration, 40 veterans, half of whom were returning from Iraq and Afghanistan conflicts participated. The participants in the study suffered from significant PTSD symptoms. The study included six weeks of music therapy in order to assess whether or not this type of therapy could lessen symptoms of PTSD. The veterans received both individual and group instructions in guitar training. The results of the study yielded positive results. The interventions helped to not only reduce symptoms of PTSD, but music therapy also lessened depressive symptoms in the veterans and improved their physical health and the quality of their lives (Sorensen, 2015).

Music therapy holds promise as a therapeutic approach for PTSD. However, more research is needed in the general population. There is even less research available on its effectiveness for use among individuals with intellectual disabilities and histories of trauma. However, since it does not rely heavily on verbal skills, it may be particularly useful for individuals whose cognitive functioning abilities lie within the lower ranges (i.e., profound and severe ID).

Pharmacological Interventions

From a biological perspective, pharmacological interventions can be used to address the dysregulation in the nervous system (i.e., in the noradrenergic and serotonergic neurotransmitter systems) that can occur in PTSD (Focht-New et al., 2008; McCarthy, 2001) in order to better manage the symptoms. Medications can help manage and lessen the physical and neurobiological changes that can occur, particularly if the PTSD symptoms are severe. They can help to reduce the symptoms (Cukor, Spitalnick, Difede, Rizzo, & Rothbaum, 2009).

Psychotropic medications that have been used as the first line of treatment due to their lower side effect profiles have included the serotonergic antidepressants known as selective serotonin reuptake inhibitors, otherwise referred to as SSRIs (Focht-New et al., 2008). Among this class of antidepressant medications, Zoloft, Paxil, Prozac, and Celexa have been used. Zoloft and Paxil have been approved by the Food and Drug Administration specifically for use with PTSD (Brady et al., 2000, Marshall et al, 2001). Another class of antidepressants known as SNRIs (serotonin-norepinephrine reuptake inhibitors) has also been used such as Venlafaxine (Effexor). Other medications to treat PTSD symptoms have included antihypertensive medications such as Clonidine and Propranolol. However, their use in treating this disorder is considered to be an "off label" use. These medications can help to lessen the physical symptoms of heightened arousal among individuals suffering from PTSD. Anti-anxiety medications (i.e., benzodiazepines) have also been used to treat severe anxiety which accompanies PTSD. However, these medications are generally used for short periods of time due to their potential for abuse. In addition, atypical antipsychotic medications have been prescribed for individuals with PTSD but are typically given to people who also experience psychotic symptoms and/or have a co-existing diagnosis of schizophrenia. Atypical antipsychotic medications have also been used to target periods of extreme agitation, anxiety, and aggression. However, the Veterans Administration and Department of Defense PTSD Clinical Practice Guidelines regarding their use states they are not recommended as monotherapy for the treatment of PTSD, but they are recommending their use if the individual is experiencing co-occurring psychotic symptoms and mood disorders.

If an individual suffers from insomnia and nightmares, Prazosin (Minipress) has been used. However, it has not specifically been approved for the treatment of PTSD by the Food and Drug Administration, but it has been used as a second line agent. It has been approved by the U.S. Food and Drug Administration to treat high blood pressure. However, its off-label use for the treatment of trauma based nightmares has been supported by the literature. There has been some research among military personnel to suggest that it may also reduce other symptoms of PTSD which individuals may experience during the day, in addition to addressing the insomnia and nightmares (Kung, Espinel, & Lapid, 2012).

Although there have been studies documenting the effectiveness of the use of these medications among individuals suffering from PTSD, empirical studies are lacking with regard to the use of these medications with individuals with intellectual disabilities and PTSD. The use of pharmacological interventions among this population is based on the effectiveness that has been demonstrated among the general population. More studies are needed regarding the effectiveness of their use among this specific population., Due to the frequency of health conditions among this population, if psychotropic medications are used as part of a treatment approach to treat PTSD among individuals with intellectual disabilities, it is important to ensure that any medical contributors or medical conditions are ruled out that could also be contributing to the symptoms (Ryan, 1994).

BASIC SUPPORTIVE APPROACHES FOR MANAGING TRAUMA-BASED REACTIONS AMONG INDIVIDUALS WITH INTELLECTUAL DISABILITIES

The therapies to address PTSD and trauma-based reactions in individuals discussed thus far have been very specific therapies which are provided by licensed mental health professionals or specifically trained individuals. The following strategies focus on some basic supportive approaches which can also be used by care providers to promote and facilitate a healing environment for individuals with intellectual disabilities and trauma histories. They can assist with re-establishing a sense of safety and lessen fear which are important in order to promote healing from trauma.

- Help the individual establish routines and schedules. Having a daily routine adds predictability. Where there is predictability, there is a greater sense of safety. However, it is important to avoid creating a schedule that is too demanding, coercive in any way, or too rigid. The schedule should include pleasurable activities for the individual. For individuals who are non-verbal, it may be helpful to create a visual schedule depicting activities and people they will be encountering that day. Sometimes a visual schedule is even useful for individuals who are verbal, since it serves as a reminder of the day's events, particularly if the individual may have some memory difficulties.

- It is important for the person to live in a safe environment. Healing is going to be hampered if the person is living in a chaotic environment and in the midst of chaotic relationships. Stability in their relationships and peace in the home is important. The person should also have a safe place to go to in order relax and recharge. Not only should the environment be safe, but it is also nice to have a "safe place" even within that environment. Having a safe environment is one of the most important elements needed to facilitate healing. For example, if the individual was emotionally abused by care providers, having the person move into a group home where clients are disruptive and frequently yelling, is going to be counterproductive and a potential obstacle to healing.
- Be aware of environments that may produce trauma triggers. For example, if the individual is in a loud and crowded area, it may trigger traumatic memories. Try to identify, prevent, lessen, or remove the triggers, when possible. For example, if an individual was in an abusive relationship, living in a home where there is yelling can serve as a trigger for memories of the past abuse. Healing cannot occur in the midst of repeated trauma or repeated activations of traumatic memories. It is important to try and eliminate as many of the frightening cues as possible.
- If the individual is verbal, he or she may need to talk about what has happened, and the person may need to do this numerous times. Avoid being judgmental or appearing shocked by the information. Often individuals who have experienced trauma are going to be looking for your reaction. If they get a negative reaction, or if they think you may not be able to handle what is being said, they may stop talking.
- It is extremely important that the individual has a sense of control over his or her life. The issue of control becomes a very critical theme for individuals who have been traumatized. Events occurred that were out of their control which can create a sense of helplessness and anxiety. Whenever possible, it is important for the individual to have choices. The more control the person has in his or her world, the better. All too often, individuals with developmental disabilities have little say or little control over the events in their lives. They may not have a choice in living arrangements, regarding who supports them on a daily basis, or where they attend a day program, etc. Providing choices over even small events or situations can be helpful. This could include providing simple choices such as asking them when they want to take a shower or make their bed. However, sometimes being presented with too many choices can be overwhelming. Therefore, this requires an additional sensitivity on the part of the care providers. Sometimes efforts that are too zealous in providing freedom of choice can be overwhelming to individuals who are not used to

having such freedoms or who lack the skills to manage such freedoms. In such cases, gradually introducing more freedoms, while teaching them any necessary skills to obtain greater future independence, may be the most beneficial approach. Also, initially providing limited choices such as asking if he or she wants to make the bed before or after breakfast may be an effective start (i.e., providing a forced choice).

- Avoid physically touching someone who has a history of sexual or physical abuse unless you have their permission to do so, or unless it is absolutely necessary to ensure their safety. Asking permission can also extend to asking permission to spend time with him or her. For example, "May I sit down with you and look at that book?" Don't force. Enough has been forced upon the person already. It is important to be sensitive to this dynamic. Don't push.
- If sleep difficulties are present, ensure that the environment is comfortable and conducive to sleep. Be careful about alarming or startling someone when you wake them up, particularly if they have had a history of being abused. Sometimes sexual abuse can occur at night making the person feel more vulnerable when they go to sleep.
- Exercise can help individuals to feel better both physically and emotionally. Exercise can reduce the level of stress produced by the body. It can stimulate endorphins which are the chemicals in the brain responsible for remediating pain, and exercise can reduce such stress hormones as cortisol and adrenaline.
- It is very important for anyone who is supporting an individual with an intellectual disability and trauma history to pay attention to the person's verbal as well as non-verbal language. When talking with the person, especially when trying to de-escalate a situation, avoid using a loud tone of voice. This may only serve to escalate the situation, since the person may have been exposed to yelling and screaming in the past. Harsh voice intonations may only serve to escalate the person's anger or anxiety. Do not allow fear or anger to be reflected in your voice tone. Firm boundaries and limits can be set using a calm tone of voice.
- Help them build their self-esteem. Build on their strengths. Help them discover activities or hobbies that they can enjoy and even develop a sense of mastery over. This will provide them with opportunities to feel good about their accomplishments.
- If you suspect someone is reacting to something that occurred years ago and the person is not in the present moment (i.e., the person has begun to dissociate or is having a flashback), try to help them ground themselves. Grounding involves helping them to stay in the here and now so that they are responding to what is occurring in the current environment. This can be accomplished in a variety of ways. For example, talk to the person about something that is happening in the here and now. Distract them with something that is immediately available in the environment.
- The importance of building positive relationships in the healing of trauma cannot be overstated. Individuals who have been traumatized can lose their sense of trust in people, particularly if the nature of the trauma consisted of

abuse at the hands of another. Trusting others can be a struggle. What is critical to restoring the ability to trust others is ensuring that the individuals who support the person are able to be consistent, reliable, patient, not reactive, calm, and not coercive in their approaches. One of the reasons why doing trauma work as a clinician, or providing care to traumatized individuals with intellectual disabilities, is so difficult is because it can take a long time to develop the trust. The individual's reactions may be out of proportion to the situation and may result in a highly reactive response on their part. For example, the individual may become verbally aggressive and even engage in aggressive or self- abusive behaviors. Do not take these behaviors personally. Your own reactions need to be tempered so that a safe environment can be created and any identifiable trauma triggers removed. The sincerity and patience of the care provider or clinician may also be tested. For example, if an abused adolescent with a mild intellectual disability is used to being rejected from a variety of foster homes, including having sustained abuse at the hands of biological parents, the person may mistrust adults. He or she may expect that this abuse and rejection will occur again. The world can feel unsafe. Remember, schemas or belief systems can develop out of trauma (such as people can't be trusted and the world is unsafe). Consequently, they may test the dedication or devotion of the very individuals who are now trying to help them. They may actually engage in behaviors meant to push others away, and if they are successful in doing this it only serves to reinforce their already existing belief that people cannot be trusted. They may not look at how their own behaviors resulted in this occurring in a type of self-fulfilling prophecy. In addition, an individual with an extensive abuse history may even have difficulty being treated well because it is so foreign to them and they are not used to it. This can be very difficult to understand for caregivers, such as foster parents, who are trying to do their best to provide a loving home for the individual. Love does not heal all wounds. Other factors need to be present such as consistency, reliability, and patience, etc. In this case, slow and steady may help to win the race. As stated previously, it is important to avoid making any promises you cannot keep. If you are not sure you can follow through with a commitment to the individual, do not make the promise or commitment. This will only serve to reinforce the belief that people can't be trusted which is a belief that can be born out of trauma. Consistency helps to build trust. Inconsistency can help destroy it. Remember: be reliable, be consistent, be calm, and establish healthy boundaries.

- If the individual is verbal, he or she may start to talk about what happened in the past. As trust begins to develop, it may prompt greater disclosure about the traumatic events. Allow the story to be told. However, individuals with PTSD may also watch for the listeners' reactions. If a reaction of disapproval or a strong emotional reaction is given, or even communicated through body language, the person may stop talking about it. It may be important for the person to safely be able to tell their story so that those experiences can be processed and worked through. If you are directly supporting the individual as a caretaker, pass on this information to a treating therapist if one is involved in the person's support plan. However, there are some who may not want to tell their story. To do so would be very overwhelming to them. Don't force disclosure in those situations.

- In the event of unresolved grief reactions resulting from the death of a significant person in the family, family interventions may be helpful. This could include the use of rituals or celebrations that perhaps mark significant events in the deceased individual's life or involve other celebratory behaviors honoring the deceased. This could help to validate and acknowledge the loss as well as provide a collective way for family members to do grief work. It can help to reduce the sense of being alone. Sometimes individuals with developmental disabilities are left out of the circle of collective grief because of concerns that they may not understand or because others may want to spare them the pain. This can leave the individual confused and alone. The person may have difficulty understanding why all of a sudden someone so important in their life is gone. Further family contacts that help affirm their connection to others who are also important to that person are also helpful. Throughout the literature on stress management there are myriads of references that discuss how important social support is in lessening life's stressors. Facilitating visits with remaining family members can be very important in strengthening a sense of feeling connected. If the individual with a developmental disability does not have contact with any family members, the support network of caretakers can also provide support. Perhaps they can locate pictures of the deceased for the bereaved and put an album together for them to be able to reminisce. However, this should also be done cautiously so as to not overwhelm the individual with emotions that may prove challenging to absorb. Therefore, experimenting and introducing these interventions at a very slow and measured pace will help to provide information as to whether or not this strategy is effective in facilitating the person's healing.

INTERVENTIONS FOR SPECIFIC TRAUMA-BASED OR STRESS-INDUCED BEHAVIORS

Some of the specific therapies which have been previously discussed should be conducted by licensed mental health professionals. However, for persons who are in the position of supporting individuals with challenging behaviors and symptoms of PTSD (or even symptoms of sub-threshold PTSD), the following are some recommendations to address some of the behavioral challenges or symptoms they may be exhibiting:

Sleep Disturbances

Individuals who have experienced trauma or trauma related stress may suffer from sleep disturbances. This can occur in the form of experiencing difficulty falling asleep or maintaining it, or both. Nightmares have been identified as a hallmark symptom of PTSD. The individual may have difficulty falling asleep because of the hypervigilance which can occur with PTSD or due to worrisome thoughts or negative thoughts. The person may feel unsafe and be plagued with worry that something bad is going to happen. If the individual is using alcohol prior to sleep it may help to facilitate falling asleep, but it can negatively impact the quality of sleep. There may also be medical issues that were associated with the trauma. For example, if someone was in a car accident he or she may be experiencing chronic pain issues which can interfere with sleep.

There are several treatments for sleep disturbances including adhering to good sleep hygiene practices, using relaxation strategies to decrease arousal, the use of medication, and improved nutrition. The following interventions are focused on improving sleep hygiene. The term "sleep hygiene" refers to incorporating or adhering to habits and practices that are conducive to sleep. Since sleep deprivation can exacerbate any physical illness as well as any psychiatric disorder, sleep is a critical component to staying healthy, both physically and mentally. The importance of obtaining quality sleep cannot be underestimated. Care providers who support individuals with intellectual disabilities can assist in their recovery process of healing from trauma by helping the individual to establish some healthy sleeping habits. For individuals with intellectual disabilities who are experiencing sleep disturbances due to PTSD or trauma-related stress, the following are recommendations to facilitate good sleep hygiene:

- Help the person to establish bedtime rituals and routines. These bedtime routines can be very simple ones. Doing the same thing every day prior to going to bed will help serve as a signal to the body and to the brain that it is time to get ready for sleep. Try to avoid naps during the day, but if a nap is necessary, ensure it is brief.
- Have the individual engage in calming activities 1-2 hours before going to bed. This could include listening to soft music, taking a long and relaxing bath, reading or looking at magazines. Encourage the person to avoid any exposure to activities that may leave the individual in a heightened level or state such as watching an action movie or a horror movie. Activities in the evening, a few hours prior to bed, should be calming activities.
- It is helpful to establish a set wake-up time daily, and it is also important to adhere to this routine on weekends. When people choose to use weekends to sleep in, it can interfere with the sleep rhythms. If the individual wishes to sleep in on the weekends, the change should not deviate too drastically from the usual routine (i.e., 1-2 hours). Changing wake-up times can disrupt the body's routine.
- It is important to have a healthy diet. Studies have shown that diet can impact the duration and quality of sleep and that an unhealthy diet is associated with more irregular sleep patterns and shorter sleep durations (Peuhkuri, Sihvola, & Korpela, 2012). These associations have been found among children and adolescents, as well as adults (Moreira et al., 2010, Chen, Wang, & Jeng, 2006; Grandner, Kripke, Naidoo, & Langer, 2010). It is also important to avoid consuming any foods or liquids that contain caffeine prior to going to bed. It can begin to produce a stimulating effect within 15 minutes of consuming it, and it can take approximately six hours before half of the caffeine is eliminated by the body. According to a review of the literature on sleep and nutrition, Peuhkuri et al. (2012) stated that a diet that is balanced, varied, and rich in fruit, vegetables, low-fat protein, and unrefined carbohydrates has been

shown to improve sleep. Although there are some foods that have traditionally been thought of as promoting sleep, such as foods that are higher in vitamins, amino acids, tryptophan (e.g., walnuts), and calcium (e.g., mild cheese), Peuhkuri et al. (2012), noted that further studies are needed with more objective or rigorous methodologies in order to more fully understand the complex relationship between sleep and nutrition.

- Exercise during the day can also facilitate sleep. However, exercise should be avoided at least for several hours before sleep. Otherwise, it can act as a stimulant making it more difficult for the individual to sleep. It is best to engage in exercise during the day rather than wait until the early evening when it could interfere with the individual's ability to calm down and prepare for sleep.
- If the individual's television watching is interfering with his or her sleep, iIt may be beneficial to remove a television from a bedroom so that the bedroom is used only for sleep. If the person resists, it may be helpful to help him/her establish a routine of when the television will be turned off. Offer to help record favorite television programs for future viewing at a more convenient time.
- Avoid stressful events prior to bed. For example, if watching the news is upsetting, it should be avoided just prior to sleep.
- The room should be conducive to sleep. The temperature in the room should not be too hot or too cold. It should be a quiet area with no noise. It should be a comfortable and soothing place. It may also be helpful to have the furniture arranged so that the individual is able to see who comes through the door. This could help to lessen any startle response that can accompany PTSD or trauma. For some individuals with a sexual abuse history, it is not uncommon for abusers to enter into bedrooms at night. Being able to see who enters the room, as well as having a night light available, may help to make the person more comfortable and feel safe enough to sleep. It is important that the individual is sleeping in a location where he or she feels safe.
- When supporting individuals with intellectual disabilities who have lived in various living arrangements (e.g., residential treatment facilities, group homes, etc.), it is also important for care providers to be aware of the individual's prior sleeping arrangements and any traumatic events that may have occurred around sleeping. For example, if the individual lived in a congregate setting and had to share a bedroom with an aggressive peer, this could have been very anxiety provoking. The individual may have not felt safe sharing the room and been fearful of future attacks. Therefore, in order to promote this individual's health from trauma-related stress, having his or her own bedroom would be recommended. Even if the individual did not experience any traumatic or stressful events around sleeping, it is still important to know about their sleeping habits and any routines and rituals around sleeping. For example, this author received a behavioral consultation request to address sleep difficulties experienced by a resident in a group home. The individual had recently moved from living in an institution to living in a community residence. However, he had difficulty falling asleep and maintaining sleep. Since the individual was non-verbal, he was not able to verbally articulate his

wants and needs. However, he effectively communicated his need through his behaviors when he kept dragging his mattress into the living room to be near the night shift staff. The change from years of living in an institution to living in a quiet home, with only a few peers, was a difficult adjustment for him. He did not feel comfortable having his own room. Rather than advise the staff to keep bringing the mattress back into his room, it was suggested that the mattress be moved into a room with another peer with a compatible personality. He was not used to sleeping alone and the changes were uncomfortable for him. Once he had a roommate, this behavior stopped, and he slept soundly.

- If sleep hygiene strategies are ineffective and the individual is not sleeping well, the short term use of psychotropic medications may be helpful. Care providers should then consult with the individual's physician or psychiatrist. If the individual is currently taking any medications, it would also be helpful to review those with the physician to determine if any of the medications could be producing sleep disturbances. For example, some of the antidepressant medications can produce vivid dreams which may be distressing to some individuals. Others can produce insomnia.

Anger Outbursts

Outbursts of anger can range in intensity. Anger is common in PTSD and is considered one of the symptoms of hyperarousal in this condition. Several strategies can be used by care providers such as family members, group home administrators, and residential staff when supporting someone with a trauma history. Some strategies may work in some situations but are ineffective in others. The following are some basic recommendations for supporting someone on a day-to-day basis who has PTSD-related anger: (Note: These strategies are supportive in nature and should not be used in lieu of professional treatment, particularly if outbursts of anger escalate into dangerous behaviors.)

- *Self-soothing activities (i.e., comfort rituals)*
  Prior to the anger outbursts, it is helpful to identify what activities tend to be comforting or self-soothing to the individual. This has been referred to in some settings as "comfort rituals." Knowing ahead of time what can soothe the person can help those who are supporting him or her so that they can direct the individual to that activity as soon as they see the anger appearing and starting to escalate. Examples of comfort rituals may be rocking in a chair, listening to music, watching television, taking a bath, etc. Obtain a list of these by either interviewing the person, if the person is verbal, or by obtaining this information from those who know the individual the best, if the individual is non-verbal. They may have seen what activities tend to be calming for the person.
- *Physical Outlets*
  Incorporate physical exercise into the individual's daily routine or as often as possible. This will provide a physical outlet for the build-up of tension.

- *Reduce Stress*
  Try to minimize stress in the home.
- *Reduce Words*
  When a person is upset there may be a tendency for those around them to try and talk to the person more (i.e., with lectures, explanations, warning, etc.). However, a person who is angry may have difficulty processing the information. Talk less when the individual is angry and more when the person is calm.
- *Use of Distraction*
  Use distraction and diversion techniques to help the person shift focus to a subject or situation that is not anger provoking.
- *Anticipate Triggers*
  Anticipate triggers because sometimes triggers can be easily identified. Some common external triggers for individuals with PTSD may be finding themselves in situations in which they are physically confined, having to seek medical treatment, events or people related to the trauma, etc. These can result in increased reactivity. Internal triggers can consist of strong negative emotions or physical sensations that remind the person of the trauma. Come up with a plan to make the situation less stressful for the person if the triggers cannot be avoided.
- *Watch for Early Warning Signs*
  Watch for early warning signs that the person is becoming angry. For example, the individual may start to pace, clench his or her fists, or start to talk in a louder voice. Try to take measures to diffuse the situation so that it doesn't escalate. You can also ask them how you can help them.
- *Remain Calm*
  Remain calm and don't let your voice escalate, since this can escalate the situation.
- *Time-Out*
  Call a time-out if the anger continues. Identify a pre-determined signal with the person ahead of any outbursts. This can be either a word or a gesture. Use that signal when reminding the person to take a time-out. If the person refuses to do so, you can take a time-out yourself by going into another area of the house (or leaving the house if doing so does not compromise the safety of the individual). However, it is important to let that person know you will come back to the issue after a short period of time. For example, if you take a time-out for 30 minutes encourage the individual to do something different for 30 minutes. Continuing to think about the issue that triggered the anger is likely to keep the anger going. Therefore, encourage the person to do something different and to engage in a distracting activity during the time-out period and then return to the discussion 30 minutes later. If the person is still not calm, take another time-out for another pre-determined period of time.
- *Safety is a Priority*
  Safety for all is important whether the person lives in a group home, a fa-

cility, or at home. If the person does not calm down despite all attempts, you can call 911 if you fear for your safety or the safety of others. If this occurs in a family home, ensure children are in a safe place.

Aggression

Outbursts of anger can range in intensity and in some cases can escalate to aggression. Aggression can be part of the "fight or flight" response when the nervous system is dysregulated. This can result in an individual becoming aggressive in response to being confronted with a trauma trigger. A trauma trigger can be an event in the environment or some behavior on the part of another person that triggers a memory of a previous traumatic experience. This could produce an aggressive or angry response on the part of the individual which may be an overreaction or an overestimation of the potential danger in a situation. Aggression may also occur because the individual's nervous system is dysregulated, and he or she is overreacting to what is actually occurring in the environment. Aggression may also occur in response to the agitation or anxiety that can be produced by experiencing a flashback. Sometimes for individuals who have experienced a sense of helplessness and a lack of control as a result of trauma, feeling as though their freedom is being challenging or restricted can serve as a trigger. If the emotions become too intense, they can lead to aggression.

The following are some supportive strategies for care providers (e.g., family members, group home administrators, etc.) to use when supporting individuals with intellectual disabilities whose aggression may be related to trauma. However, professional help should still be sought due to the potential seriousness of this behavior:

- *Identify Trauma Triggers*
  It is important to try and prevent the chance of aggression occurring. This can be done by trying to identify any trauma triggers the person may have and trying to remove them, lessen them, or prepare for them. This comes from knowing the person's history. If the person's history is unavailable to the extent that identifying the trauma triggers can be difficult, then note if there is a theme or a set of common denominators in the situations which trigger such reactivity. For example, if the person becomes agitated and there are more frequent incidents of being aggressive when a tall male staff member with dark hair works with him, then this can help to provide clues as to the types of situations they were in previously when the trauma occurred. It is important to try and remove these types of triggers so the person can heal and a sense of safety and security can be re-established.
- *Intervene Early*
  Intervene early when the person is just starting to exhibit signs of distress. Try to determine the cause of the distress early before it escalates. For example, is the person starting to pace or making statements that indicate they are becoming fearful? Reassure the person that he or she is safe and try to remove the stimulus that is starting to make them upset if possible. If the person is becoming agitated because of being over-stimulated by the environment, lower the noise. Create a calmer and quieter environment. Listen to what the person is saying, it may provide clues to what they need.

For example, a client once became anxious at her physician's office, and she started to raise her voice. She also had a history of aggression. She began to also say, "Don't touch me." She was reassured that no one was going to touch her and that the doctor was just going to talk to her. However, we also allowed her to sit near the door rather than in the back of the room so that she did not feel confined or cornered. Asking someone who has a trauma history to wait in a closed area may be very distressing to the individual depending upon the nature of the trauma experienced. In this case, she was also given a choice, and she was asked if she would be more comfortable waiting in the waiting room and they could see if the doctor could meet with her in a larger area. This was enough to calm her down. She also noted that the doctor's nurse seemed nice so we solicited the help of the nurse to also come over and talk with her.

- *Keep Language Simple*
  When talking with the person, keep your language simple. Be concise and repeat yourself as needed. Use simple and concrete statements. Avoid a lot of verbiage. Ensure any directions that you are giving are short, clear, and direct and are delivered without a hostile or angry, reactive tone. Remember, you will not be able to gain control of the situation if you are out of control yourself. Be aware of your own reactions.

- *Respect Personal Space*
  Be respectful of personal space and keep a distance. Entering the person's physical space can escalate the situation. Sometimes it is best to keep at least a two-arm distance from the person. Increase your distance if the person appears to be paranoid or extremely fearful. If you are approaching the person, stand on their non-dominant side. For example, if the person is right handed, approach them and stand by their left side. It is particularly important to try to avoid touching an individual who is actively psychotic.

- *Avoid Provocative Language*
  Avoid the use of any language that sounds threatening or can be taken in a provocative, inflammatory, or threatening manner.

- *Set Limits as Needed*
  Set boundaries and limits as needed but do so firmly and calmly.

- *Decrease Environmental Stimulation*
  Ensure the environment is quiet and not chaotic. For example, if a television is playing loudly in the background or if there is music and it is overstimulating, either lower the volume or shut off the devices.

- *Avoid Overwhelming the Person*
  It is important to not overwhelm the person. Having several people trying to support the individual and de-escalate the situation may prove to be too much for that person. It may be best to have one or two people dealing with the individual at a time. However, this does not mean that other people are not in the background for assistance, if needed. It is never wise to approach an angry, agitated individual alone.

- *Avoid Sudden Movements*
  Avoid making any quick or sudden movements and do not turn your back on someone who is angry. It is important to be able to monitor their movements.
- *Avoid Staring*
  Avoid any eye contact that is glaring or staring.
- *Scan the Environment*
  Scan the environment to ensure that any objects that could be used as weapons are removed.
- *Maintain a Non-Threatening Posture*
  Ensure that your posture is non-threatening. Maintain a calm demeanor.
- *Assess for Needs*
  Ask the person what they need to feel safe.
- *Seek Psychiatric Assistance*
  If these episodes are severe enough to present a danger to others or to the person themselves, consult with a psychiatrist for a medication evaluation. Again, properly used and monitored, psychotropic medications can help to lessen the individual's distress and reactivity.
- *Maintain a Calm Demeanor*
  Remember: Being calm can have a contagious effect the same way that fear can. Remain calm. Watch your body language so that you do not unintentionally escalate the situation. Maintain a neutral facial expression. If you yourself are stressed and nervous, watch your breathing. Control your breathing.
- *Maintain an Escape Route*
  Maintain an escape route for both you and the person. Don't get yourself cornered in a small contained area and don't corner the person. If in danger, call 911.

MEDICAL TRAUMA - FEARFULNESS WITH MEDICAL EXAMINATIONS AND PROCEDURES

The aftereffects of medical assessments, interventions, and procedures can produce symptoms of depression, anxiety, and traumatic stress responses (Hall & Hall, 2013). Medical trauma can also result in symptoms of posttraumatic stress disorder or sub-threshold presentations of PTSD. It can also exacerbate any existing psychiatric conditions or re-awaken past symptoms of PTSD (Babbel, 2011).

Medical procedures are often overlooked when considering potential sources of trauma or trauma-based reactions. Undergoing medical procedures or examinations can be anxiety provoking, distressing, and even frightening for individuals in the general population even if the procedures are not highly invasive or posing a physical threat (O'Hare, Ghoneim, Himrichs, Mehta, & Wright, 1989). Allen and Kupzyk (2016) noted that non-compliance with medical procedures in the general population is often fear based. Consequently, imagine the impact that medical procedures or assessments can have on individuals with intellectual disabilities who often have little or no control over attending the appointments or even consenting to the procedures. There have been studies which have also shown that individuals with developmental disabilities, particularly those with autism, have experienced more fears and anxieties around medical procedures when compared to the general population (Gillis, Hammond Natof, Lockshin, & Romanczyk, 2009; Knapp, Barrett, Groden, & Groden, 1992). Therefore, addressing any anxieties and assessing for past traumatic experiences is very important in ensuring the individual's cooperation for future medical appointments and clinics. It is especially important if you consider that there are over 300 different syndromes that can cause developmental disabilities and specific medical issues can occur as a result of some of these syndromes. Consequently, more frequent medical monitoring and interventions may be required.

Fearfulness or past traumas around medical visits and procedures can result in individuals with developmental disabilities becoming resistive and sometimes even aggression towards both their care takers and medical personnel. They may even engage in property destruction while in the doctor's office out of anxiety or out of a desperate effort to escape an anxiety provoking situation. Therefore, when supporting individuals with intellectual disabilities it is important to obtain information regarding their history with regard to their cooperation with medical appointments and the behaviors that they have exhibited during past appointments. This will help to ensure that any distress or anxieties are addressed in order to maintain their health and safety, as well as the safety of medical personnel who will be meeting with them. There are some basic strategies that may help to lessen the anxiety, as well as some strategies that may require more intensive professional assistance. The following are some basic supportive strategies that can be used to help lessen distress or anxiety around medical appointments:

- If an individual has a history of experiencing anxiety and resistance over visits, it can be helpful to have familiar and trusted staff or trusted significant others accompany the individual.
- Familiarizing the person with the office and the office staff can also be helpful. Planning multiple, short, and positive visits to the office can be helpful prior to the actual day of the appointment. (If this produces too much anxiety, then a more formal de-sensitization protocol may need to be introduced by a licensed mental health professional.) These "field trips" can also be associated with other positive trips. For example, after visiting the doctor's office, there is a visit to the local ice cream store.
- Explain to the individual what is happening, or going to happen, with reassurance that he or she is safe.
- Sometimes waiting in the waiting room can be distressing, since it is a new environment with new sights and sounds. Therefore, waiting in the car until the actual appointment can lessen anxiety for some people. The caretaker can check in by phone, or another care provider, who may also be attending, can check in with the receptionist until the actual appointment time. Consequently, when the doctor is ready to see the individual the person can immediately go into the office and be seen. This can be particularly helpful if the waiting room is busy. Some individuals with intellectual disabilities (particularly if there is an additional diagnosis of autism) are sensitive to a lot of

environmental noise and stimulation, and waiting in the waiting room can be difficult. If it is not possible or advisable to remain in the car, and the waiting room is crowded, overstimulating, or confining, wait in another area, if one can be located that is quieter and less confined. However, be careful that the person is not near a door so that if they quickly tried to exit they would find themselves running into a parking lot or into the street. It is also important never to leave the person you are supporting alone in the car or unsupervised during such times. This is why it is important to have two people attending the appointment, if possible, particularly when supporting someone with ID who has been known to be anxious and/or uncooperative around medical appointments.

- When possible, park as close to the building and office as possible. This will allow for quick entrances and exits.
- Providing distractions while waiting can also help to lessen anxiety. This could include activities that they enjoy such as looking at certain magazines or looking at pictures on an iPad. It can be helpful if the care providers bring some of the individual's preferred items or activities to the appointments.
- It is important to observe for early signs of agitation and increased anxiety. For example, if the person is verbal, they may be directly or indirectly communicate their growing discomfort or distress. If they are not able to verbally communicate distress, watch for non-verbal warning signs of confusion or distress. For example, the person may become more restless, or his or her facial expression may become tense. Upon seeing early warning signs, explain to them what is happening, reassure them, and if possible, make any environmental modifications that may help to lessen their anxiety.
- Remain calm and maintain a demeanor of calmness in order to avoid any contagion effect of anxiety. If you are anxious, the individual you are supporting may sense that, and it can add to his or her distress.
- Encourage the doctor or other medical personnel to use a gentle approach. They may even demonstrate something as simple as taking a blood pressure reading on you so that you can show the person that nothing bad is going to happen to them.
- Try to schedule the appointments either as the first appointment of the morning, so that the doctor is not rushed and the waiting room is not too crowded, or as the last appointment of the day. However, the last appointment of the day increases the risk of a longer wait time because the doctor may have fallen behind in the schedule.
- After the medical appointment, have either a rewarding activity available or a pleasurable activity scheduled. This will help to facilitate a more positive association with doctors' appointments. Try to have the visits end on a positive note.
- It is also important to obtain a medication sedation history that has been used for prior medical appointments and/or procedures. For example, has the individual ever required medication to help alleviate any anxiety? What was that medication and its dosage, and was it effective or did the person require MAC sedation (i.e., monitored anesthesia care)? If necessary, the individual may

need to see a psychiatrist or family physician in order to obtain a prescription for some form of a sedative, if the individual has been too anxious and uncooperative in the past over medical appointments or procedures. If possible, finding a mobile physician service or a mobile lab (that does blood draws) that can come to the home can help to create a less threatening experience. With the assistance of a behavior specialist or mental health professional, a desensitization program can also be written and implemented to help lessen anxiety for the individual. This would involve gradually exposing the individual to aspects of the feared situation but doing so very slowly and over repeated trials, gradually increasing the exposure. A desensitization hierarchy would be constructed so that each step in the process is broken down into incremental steps. The person does not progress to the next step until he or she does not experience anxiety at that particular step.

The Family Environment and Support Social Network

It is important that parents or other support people are informed and educated about the possible signs and symptoms of traumatic stress reactions and PTSD, if they are providing care and support for their relatives with intellectual disabilities and trauma histories. This is particularly important since individuals with ID are usually dependent upon their caretakers for so many of their needs. Educating significant people in the person's support network is important if the individual is exhibiting problematic behaviors that prove to be very challenging to the family or for his or her support network. For example, if an individual with ID is responding to trauma with outbursts of anger or aggressive behavior, this can be extremely difficult on their support system. Helping the individual's support network to understand the possible origins of the behavior may also make it easier to manage. Understanding may encourage empathy. Educating parents and other members of the individual's support system is also important in order to ensure the removal of trauma triggers and to help ensure that a safe environment is created. For example, if an individual with ID was emotionally and/or physically abused by a previous caretaker, and if the parent responds with a loud and threatening voice in response to the person's behaviors, it can exacerbate the situation, and the situation could escalate. It is also important to be sensitive to family members in discussing PTSD, since they themselves may have been diagnosed with it or have been the victims of abuse. They may also be experiencing guilt about not having been able to prevent the trauma and protect their loved one. Having a loved one suffer from PTSD can change the dynamics of a family requiring support for all.

Chapter 8

Individual Stories/Case Studies

When behavior analysts are asked to intervene to address challenging behaviors among individuals with intellectual disabilities, they approach situations with specific strategies and several standard procedures. The result is a systematic and comprehensive analysis of the behaviors often referred to as a functional behavioral assessment. This assessment involves the use of different methods necessary to determine why a specific challenging behavior is occurring. Assessment methods may include information that is obtained from a variety of sources, both direct and indirect, such as directly observing the individual, interviewing people who support the person, reviewing available records, and interviewing the individual directly, if he or she possesses verbal skills. Information can also be obtained by administering questionnaires, rating scales, or standardized tests. In addition, information is collected by conducting a functional analysis. When conducting a functional analysis, a behavioral consultant attempts to determine why a behavior is occurring and to identify cause and effect (i.e., environment-behavior) relationships. In this type of analysis, the analyst is looking at specific conditions which occurred just prior to the behavior being exhibited, the consequences of the behavior, and any contingencies which occurred. If the factors can be identified that are causing and maintaining the behaviors, then future situations can be manipulated or changed in order to produce a change in behaviors. It is assumed that if the function of the maladaptive behavior can be identified (with the function serving some need for the individual) then the individual can be taught other more adaptive and effective ways to meet his or her needs. This type of functional analysis is a common practice in the field of behavioral analysis (Iwata & Dozier, 2008).

It is also important to adopt a holistic approach when analyzing behaviors. Such an approach considers the possibility that an individual's behavior may be caused or influenced by factors beyond the individual's control and may not be maladaptive in nature. As an example, it is important to rule out (or rule in) any medical causes for the behavioral challenges. As part of the analysis, it is also important to ensure that any underlying psychiatric issues which may be causing or contributing to the behavioral challenges are also identified and treated such as an anxiety or depressive disorder. After considering these two possibilities (medical and psychiatric), consideration is given to whether the maladaptive behavior is a learned behavior reinforced by certain contingencies or consequences. However, consider another element to this analysis, another lens from which to view the behaviors, and that lens includes adopting a trauma-informed perspective in the assessment process.

By introducing a trauma-sensitive framework, the analysis now includes assessing for trauma in the person's history and the impact traumatic experiences may have on the person's current behaviors and functioning. This changes the clinician's perspective from one of asking, "What is wrong with John?" to "What happened to John?" Trauma assessment then becomes one of the initial steps in the behavioral analysis which explores the impact that traumatic events may be having on the individual's behaviors. Treatment of the trauma and trauma-sensitive interventions are then incorporated into the overall treatment plan. Adhering to a trauma-informed or trauma-sensitive approach also focuses on promoting a healing environment for the individual. Identifying any current sources of trauma, removing trauma triggers, and treating the emotional and physical sequelae of past traumas may facilitate the individual's healing. This in turn may help to reduce or eliminate any challenging behaviors, if those behaviors were trauma induced. There are many situations when individuals with severe behavioral reputations have not responded to behavioral interventions or other types of supports and approaches. In these types of situations, it may be that the challenging behaviors had their origins in trauma, and as these traumatic origins or roots were overlooked it rendered the interventions ineffective.

How to Incorporate a Trauma Sensitive Approach into the Analysis of Behaviors

How can a trauma-sensitive perspective be introduced when analyzing the possible causes of challenging behaviors among individuals with intellectual disabilities? The following are suggested methods for not only assessing for trauma but also incorporating the findings into a comprehensive approach aimed at addressing behavioral challenges:

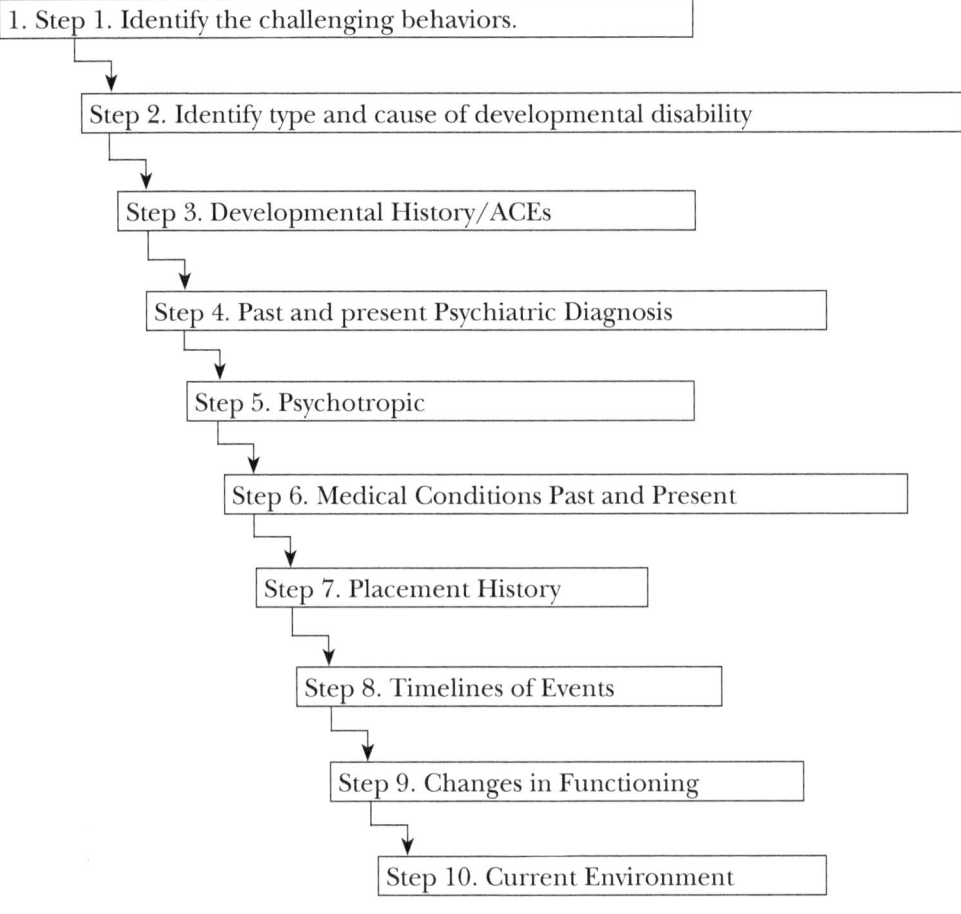

Step 1. Identify the Challenging Behaviors

Identify aspects of the behavior that include the following variables: what, when, where, and with whom. What does the behavior look like? When does it occur? Where and with whom does it occur? This is part of conducting a functional analysis. By determining the *what, when, where* and *with whom* conditions under which the behaviors occur (and the consequences of those behaviors), it is possible to theorize about the functions served by behavior(s) (e.g., avoidance, tension reduction, etc.). For example, if the behavior only occurs with the individual's mother, and it only occurs when she asks him to make his bed, then perhaps it is his way of avoiding the task as he knows his avoidance tactics may be successful with her.

Step 2. Identify the Type and Cause of the Developmental Disability

Identify the type of developmental disability (i.e., autism, intellectual disability, and the severity of the intellectual disability). If possible, find out the cause of the developmental disability. It may be in the records, or it may never have been identified. This information becomes important if the developmental disability was caused by a syndrome, as syndromes may have certain medical conditions associated with them. Certain syndromes may also have specific behaviors or behavioral characteristics attributed to the syndrome as well. This is referred to as a behavioral phenotype.

Step 3. Developmental History/ACEs

A developmental history includes information regarding potentially significant and historical events or milestones during an individual's childhood. Typically it includes information regarding his or her birth (including any complications) and developmental milestones such as the time when he or she began walking, talking, etc. Since the first tenet of trauma-informed work is to explore the person's history for the presence of any possible traumas, included in this section is also whether a history of abuse, neglect, or other adverse childhood experiences exists. The identification of adverse childhood events may help to determine if some of individual's behaviors are the result of traumatic experiences, particularly given the impact early childhood experiences can have on behavior in adulthood. Such adverse experiences can also include relationship losses, changes in residences including out-of-home placements, health crises, and exposure to violence, etc.

Step 4. Past and Present Psychiatric Diagnoses

Along with the developmental disability, has the individual ever exhibited any behaviors that have been attributable to a psychiatric condition such as anxiety or depression? For example, if an individual does not want to leave the house, is it due to a possible anxiety disorder? Identifying both current and past psychiatric diagnoses is helpful in determining whether the behavior is symptomatic of a current psychiatric condition or if a past psychiatric condition is re-emerging. Is there a current diagnosis of PTSD, a past diagnosis of PTSD, or a rule out of PTSD in the person's record?

Step 5. Psychotropic Medications

It is important to obtain information on the types of medication the individual is receiving. This would include any psychotropic medications (i.e., medications given for any psychiatric conditions or used to address any significant behavioral challenges) as well as any medications prescribed for medical conditions. Medications can cause side effects which can impact behavior. It is also extremely helpful to obtain a psychotropic medication history which includes any medication successes or failures and their corresponding dosages. Were there any medications which caused severe side effects that may have precipitated a health crisis and been traumatic for the individual?

Step 6. Medical Conditions Past and Present

Obtain information regarding the person's medical conditions. As an initial step it is important to rule out any medical contributors that could be influencing or contributing to the individual's behavioral challenges. It is also helpful to obtain a medical history should any past medical issues resurface, particularly in the case of medical conditions which can be reoccurring. Note whether or not the individual has had any major changes in health status that could be stressful. Medical procedures can also be traumatic for some individuals, particularly if they are invasive. Were there any medical conditions that exist or existed as a result of any traumatic events?

Step 7. Placement History

It is important to gather information about the person's current living situation, but it is also important to gather information about past living arrangements. Obtaining a placement history can provide a wealth of information, and, in particular, it can provide clues to possible traumas. A placement history helps to construct a timeline of the individual's life. How long has the person lived in each residence and/or facility and what reasons did he or she have for leaving? A history of numerous placements, including the types of placements, could signal a variety of losses and traumatic events such as psychiatric hospitalizations, loss of friendships, relationships, separation from family members, and police interventions due to dangerous behaviors, etc. As an example, if an out-of-home placement occurred as a child, it may have been due to abuse (if the placement was the result of CPS investigations or court involvement). This would clearly speak to early childhood traumas or early adverse events.

Has the person had a history of numerous psychiatric hospitalizations, time spent in jail, or a history of living in institutions? Trauma from being incarcerated, being restrained, and living in settings where other may be exhibiting dangerous behaviors may be part of the individual's history.

Step 8. Timeline of Events

It can be very informative to explore a timeline of events in a person's life and to place the behaviors within the context of that history. This timeline can also be superimposed upon the placement timeline identified in step 7. This would include noting how long the behaviors have been occurring. Do the behaviors have an acute onset or are they long-standing behaviors? Look at the environments in which the behaviors occur. Do the behaviors bear any resemblance to any of the symptom clusters of PTSD (e.g., avoidance behaviors, alternations in reactivity or arousal, marked alterations in cognition or mood, or intrusive symptoms, etc.)? By constructing a timeline of events in the person's history, it becomes easier to identify potential sources of stress or trauma. (The questions in the questionnaires presented in Chapter 4 could be used as a foundation for identifying potential sources of traumatic experiences.)

Step 9. Changes in Functioning

Have there been any changes in the person's level of functioning since experiencing the events identified on the timelines? Were any of these events associated with any behavioral changes? If there was trauma, was it the result of a single event or a series of events (or repeated events)? If changes in the individual's baseline functioning can be identified, it can help determine whether or not the individual has experienced any traumatic events that continue to adversely impact his or her daily life.

Step 10. Current Environment

Are there aspects of the individual's living environment or current interpersonal relationships that are serving as continued triggers for trauma-related stress reactions? Is it a safe environment (both physically and emotionally) for the person, or does the current environment continue to perpetuate fear or inhibit the person's ability to heal from past traumatic or stressful experiences? This would also include exploring the status of current interpersonal relationships and the identification of any dysfunction within the household.

The Final Analysis

Behavioral assessments which incorporate all the steps outlined, and which are tailored to an individual's cognitive level of functioning, possess a greater chance of developing effective interventions. The following case studies illustrate the use of this approach which incorporates not only assessing for traumatic events but recommendations for trauma-sensitive interventions.

John's Story

John's story is a perfect example of how adopting a trauma-informed approach can be an effective strategy in addressing challenging behaviors. John was a 28-year-old man with Down syndrome who lived in a group home (i.e., an adult residential facility) with five other people. He was diagnosed with an intellectual disability that was in the mild range as a result of the syndrome. John was non-verbal, but he did know a few signs (i.e., American Sign Language), and he had no visual or hearing deficits identified. John also did not have a psychiatric diagnosis at the time of the referral, but he had a past diagnosis of adjustment disorder with depressed mood. He received that diagnosis after he had moved out of his family home and into his first group home years ago.

At the time of the behavioral consultation request, John had been living in a community residence with five other clients for a little less than a year. During that time he had two brief psychiatric hospitalizations for aggression. His behavioral challenges included not only aggression, but frequent refusals to listen to the staff, increased sleeping, increased resistance to leaving the house, and intermittent incidents of bedwetting. John was beginning to spend more time in his room, alone and isolated. Incidents of property destruction were infrequent and occurred approximately four times within a ten month period. The biggest concern was his aggression towards the staff and towards his mother who would visit intermittently. When he was aggressive, staff stated the incidents of hitting and punching would sometimes appear to occur "out of the blue." He was also becoming aggressive towards his peers in the home. In addition, there were a few occasions in which he was aggressive while attending some social activities out of the home. For example, he became aggressive towards a staff member while attending a social club event. However, John had recently stopped attending any activities out of the home and was becoming more resistant to leaving the residence. He was also becoming increasingly aggressive towards staff when they had to take him to doctors' appointments. John had stopped attending a day program partly due to his increasingly aggressive behavior but also because he did not want to leave the residence.

Prior to his admission to his current group home, he had been living with his younger brother, his sister-in-law, and their young daughter. His brother had to seek out-of-home placement due to John's incidents of aggression towards their daughter, as well as towards his sister-in-law. Prior to residing with his brother, John lived in another group home for approximately seven or eight years which had been his first out-of-home placement. Before his admission to that home, he had been living with his mother and brother since his birth.

After moving into his current group home, John's family did not come to visit him for several months and did not contact him. It was several months before his mother came to visit, and then she came to see him three times within a year's time. His brother accompanied their mother to see John for two of the visits. John became aggressive towards his mother at the end of each of her visits. One of his psychiatric hospitalizations occurred a few hours after one of the visits when he attacked another peer in the home following his mother's departure. For a week or so after his mother's visits John's sleeping habits would change. He would sleep for longer periods, and he would not get up until around 11:00 or noon; when he did get up he would frequently have had an incident of nighttime urinary incontinence. His physically aggressive behaviors were also increasing and were directed at both the staff and the other residents in the home. His aggression towards staff and peers in the group home had occurred even prior to his mother beginning her visits, but they were increasing.

A new peer moved into the home who was very loud and physically intrusive (i.e., stand too close to people). The new peer was very aggressive at times towards the other residents (including John), and his assaultive behavior necessitated police involvement on several occasions. During one of the times when the new resident was aggressive, the police arrived and took the peer and John to the hospital. John became highly agitated when he saw the police and gestured as though he was going to hit them. In response, the police felt John also needed to go to the psychiatric hospital for evaluation.

Because of John's history of aggressiveness towards his mother at the end of their visits, she stopped visiting him. At the time of the behavioral consultation, John had not seen her in months. However, whenever a package would come to the house, or if John saw the staff opening an envelope, he would sign the word for mother with a questioning look as his face (as if he was asking if the mail was for him). Sometimes, if the staff bought him something (such as a new shirt), they would say it was from his mother. This would produce a grin from John that staff said went from "ear to ear" and he was in a good mood for the remainder of the day.

When this author first met John, who was primarily non-verbal (other than to make a few vocalizations and use a few signs), he immediately lifted his shirt and pointed to scars on his chest near his heart which looked like surgical scars. He also had other scars on other areas of his chest and near his abdomen. While pointing, he would make various vocalizations accompanied by a slight level of agitation, but his vocalizations were indiscernible. The house manager stated this was typical for John to do when he met new people but this behavior was not given any significance. According to the staff, it was just something John did.

Although the staff liked John, the house administrator was concerned that if the aggression did not stop, or if John's behaviors were not more manageable, he would have to leave.

The Analysis

If we use the ten steps identified in the beginning of the chapter, the following analysis unfolds:

Step 1: *Identify the Challenging Behaviors*

Aggression

John was becoming increasingly aggressive and his aggression was directed towards staff and his peers, as well as towards his family at the conclusion of their visits. It occurred across environments including in the community when he attended a social event and at home. John's history of aggression consisted of hitting people either by punching or slapping them. After carefully examining his aggression, including the situations that preceded it, the people he targeted, and the consequences of his actions, the following information was obtained:

- He was more likely to be aggressive with females and with new staff.
- He was more likely to be aggressive if someone approached him from the side, or if he was startled (and he appeared to be startled often).
- The incidents of aggression were more likely if he didn't get what he wanted for dinner or when he was not able to have certain foods he wanted.
- He was more likely to be aggressive when the house manager was not present.
- If another peer was having an emotional outburst, it increased the likelihood that John would be aggressive towards the staff.
- He could be aggressive when he attended doctors' appointments.
- John had been aggressive in new environments when there were a lot of people around him.
- He had been aggressive towards his mother at the end of their visits when she was getting ready to leave.
- When he couldn't get something he wanted, he was more likely to hit the staff.
- Staff also reported that he could be aggressive "out of the blue" when there were no readily identifiable environmental triggers.
- If he was in pain he would often become more irritable and more aggressive.

Resistance

John was also becoming increasingly more resistant to listening to the staff and cooperating with their requests. The following were some of the situations which were more likely to trigger his refusals:

- When the staff would attempt to get him to shower, change his clothes, and go on an outing, he would become more resistant.
- When asked to do a task he didn't want to do, he would not want to cooperate with the staff.
- He was becoming more resistant to attending his doctors' appointments which required more prompting and coaxing from the staff.
- After his mother would leave, he would become more resistant with the staff and this lasted sometimes for days afterwards. He would want to spend more time in bed following her visits.
- If staff tried to get him out of bed before noon or early afternoon, he would be more resistant.
- John was more resistant with the staff if the house manager was not on duty for a particular shift.

- His resistance also seemed to increase when he was having increased incidents of bedwetting.

Step 2: Identify the Type and Cause of the Developmental Disability

John was diagnosed with Down syndrome and an intellectual disability that was in the mild range. There are numerous medical conditions that can occur with that syndrome. For example, it is extremely common for individuals with this syndrome to have sleep apnea. This condition (in which respirations briefly stop at night) can lead to increased daytime fatigue and irritability and resemble depression. Cardiac issues are also common among individuals with this syndrome.

Step 3: Developmental History/ACEs

Information regarding John's placement history was sparse as his case was new to the agency serving him. His family had moved to a different county, and the records did not follow him. However, the house manager knew that John had previously resided in a group home and had previously lived with his younger brother, prior to moving into his current group home. Lacking information, this author contacted his brother who was able to provide a more complete history. John's brother stated that their mother suffered from severe depression and was not very responsive to John's needs throughout the years, since she was overwhelmed by the level of care he needed. Her struggles with severe depression made it difficult for her to care for herself at times and to even care for John's brother who did not have a developmental disability. Their father left when John was 8 years of age and had not been involved since. His whereabouts were unknown. John's brother stated that both he and John had difficult childhoods due to their mother's emotional issues, but he felt that John had received the brunt of the difficulties. He recalled his mother yelling at John on numerous occasions and hitting him, but he didn't remember John being aggressive while he lived at home. His brother also stated that their mother would often leave John in his care. There were periods of time when her mood would improve but she would have reoccurring bouts of disabling depression. If John became upset during those times, she would try to quickly calm him down by giving him whatever he wanted. Eventually, she sought out-of-home placement for John because she was unable to provide him with the care he needed. When asked about John's medical history, his brother stated he recalled John required heart surgery as a child which explained some of the scars but could not provide many additional details. He thought the surgery may have been needed to correct a heart valve.

Step 4: Past and Present Psychiatric Diagnoses

A review of John's records from the agency responsible for his placement revealed a past diagnosis of adjustment disorder with depressed mood. This diagnosis was given several months after John's first out-of-home placement from his family home. He began exhibiting behavioral issues after moving into his first group home, such as aggressive behaviors and sleep disruptions. He also became more withdrawn, would spend more time in his room, and did not want to attend various activities. This was the only diagnosis in his record. There was no current psychiatric diagnosis.

Step 5: Psychotropic Medications

The only psychotropic medication John was receiving was Risperdal, and he was receiving a moderate dosage on a daily basis. He was also receiving a stool softener due to bouts of constipation from the Risperdal.

Step 6: Medical Conditions Past and Present

As previously stated, John's brother reported that John had heart surgery as a child and could not recall many of the details beyond believing it had to do with fixing a valve in his heart.

With regard to John's current medical conditions, he was intermittently receiving trials of antibiotics for repeated urinary infections, and his incidents of bedwetting were associated with these infections. After treatment, his incidents of wetting the bed stopped but they would return when the infection returned. Staff also reported that John wanted to sleep more and spend more time in bed when he had the infections.

Step 7: Placement History

When John was approximately 18 or 19 years of age, he moved from his family home into his first group home. He lived in that group home for approximately eight years. During that time the home had several different administrators, and there were frequent changes in staffing. His brother would occasionally visit John, and he would intermittently find some wounds or bruises on his brother. When he questioned the staff, they noted the bruises were the result of John's self-abusive behavior. They stated John would intermittently punch himself when he was frustrated. However, John's brother did not recall ever seeing John being self-abusive. He began to suspect that his brother was being mistreated. He also found that on occasions when he visited John, the home was not clean and his brother had not bathed in some time. He reported his concerns about John's treatment to local agencies, but the staff member from the overseeing agency for the home assigned to the case stated that the alleged abuse could not be substantiated. John's brother was of the belief that the staff investigating the matter had also been friends with the group home administrator. His brother believed that some of the scars on John were the result of him being physical abused by either the staff or by the other residents in the home. John's brother finally decided to take John out of the home so that he could live with him and his family because of growing concerns about the care John was receiving and concerns for his safety. John's brother did not have concerns about the current group home staff. He felt they were caring and attentive.

After John went to live with his brother, John starting exhibiting aggressive behaviors towards his brother, his sister-in-law, and their two-year-old daughter. This would typically occur when they tried to introduce some demands or introduce some type of daily structure for John. He would also occasionally become aggressive for unknown reasons even when no situational trigger could be identified. Out of concern for the safety of his daughter and his wife, his brother sought out-of-home placement for John. While John lived with his brother, he rarely saw his mother. Because her depression became so disabling, his contact with her became even more infrequent once John moved into his first group home. Another group home (i.e., adult residential facility) was eventually located where John was residing at the time of the behavioral consultation referral.

Step 8: Timeline of Events

If a timeline is constructed of the events in John's life, it would include the following:
- He had a history of numerous adverse childhood events including neglect by his mother who had severe depression. Her care for him was inconsistent, and his father left the family when John was approximately 8 years of age.
- He had an out-of-home placement due to his mother's inability to care for him. After his initial admission to a group home, John became aggressive, irritable, and more withdrawn, and this resulted in him receiving a diagnosis of an adjustment disorder with depressed mood indicating he had difficulty adjusting to the change. According to his record, his behavior began to improve after several months of living in the first residence, and his aggression decreased, and he became more active. There was also a reference in the available records that stated John tended to have a very difficult time with changes and transitions.
- John may have suffered abuse and neglect while living in the first group home. His family's suspicions that he was being abused resulted in John moving into his brother's home.
- Due to behavioral challenges John was exhibiting towards his family members, including aggression and non-compliance, he had to leave and move into another group home.
- After moving into another group home (his current residence), there was an increase in John's incidents of aggression and his non-compliance. He was sleeping more, eating more, and becoming more withdrawn. He just wanted to sleep or spend time away from everyone either watching television in a separate part of the house or staying in his bedroom. He would often refuse to attend outings in the community with the staff and other peers. He was also becoming increasingly aggressive towards peers.
- After he moved into his current group home, his family did not come to visit him immediately. It was months before his mother would come to visit. His brother came to visit him on occasion, sometimes accompanying his mother. John was very aggressive with her towards the end of each of their visits when she told him it was time for her to leave. For a week or so after his mother's visits, John would sleep more and spend more time in his room.
- John had a psychiatric hospitalization after one of his mother's visits when he attacked another peer in the home. Because of John's aggressiveness, his mother stopped visiting him.
- This was followed by the introduction of a new resident to the home. Another young man was admitted who was highly aggressive towards John. During one of the altercations both John and the new resident were taken by the police to a local psychiatric hospital for screening and admission.

Step 9: Changes in Functioning

John was becoming more withdrawn, and he wanted to sleep more after his visits with his mother. The only time the staff found him to be cheerful and more engaged is when a package came to the house and he thought it was from his mother. In order to cheer him up, the staff would sometimes tell him he received something from her and give him an item that he thought was bought by her. Staff said this would make him smile from "ear to ear." He was becoming increasing more withdrawn, more irritable, and more aggressive. His records also indicated that he had difficulties adjusting after his first move out of his family residence. His difficulties adjusting at that time in his life, and with the changes he was experiencing, warranted a diagnosis of an adjustment disorder.

Step 10: Current Environment

Staff was fond of John, and they were trying to do their best to manage his behaviors. The other residents had not been aggressive towards him or towards the staff with the exception of the one peer who just recently moved into the home. On occasion, he would target John and become aggressive towards him. Otherwise, the house was relatively quiet, and the other residents were not exhibiting significant behavioral challenges.

The Final Analysis – Putting it All Together

It is important when addressing John's challenging behaviors to consider all of the following in the final analysis:
1. Are there any medical contributors to his behavior challenges?
2. Are there any psychiatric conditions that are either causing or influencing his behaviors? This could include an anxiety or depressive disorder, PTSD, or even sub-threshold PTSD symptoms.
3. Are any of these behaviors learned? For example, is he aggressive because prior experiences have taught him that such behavior allows him to get something he wants or escape a task that he doesn't want to do?

Initially, it is important to assess whether or not the behavioral challenges are the result of medical, psychiatric, or learned behaviors. This information can then be combined with the other information obtained in each of the 10 steps leading to the final analysis. It leads to several hypotheses about why the behaviors are occurring. From this vantage point, interventions can then be formulated.

With regard to the medical rule outs, John's was seen by a urologist who conducted an ultrasound and found that John had a problem with fully emptying his bladder. Further medical consultations were being scheduled. Periodic urinalyses were being conducted by the physician to ensure John did not have another urinary tract infection. It was also thought that the medication, Risperdal, may have been predisposing him to have urinary tract infections. This was being discussed with both the urologist and with John's psychiatrist. Because John was also very fatigued and hard to awaken in the morning, his physician thought he may also be suffering from sleep apnea, given the increased prevalence of this condition among individuals with Down syndrome. However, in order to determine if John did in fact have this condition, it would require a sleep study. John's physician (as well as the staff) did not believe John would cooperate with the study, and even if he did, they did not believe John would be receptive to wearing a mask at night to treat it.

With regard to any psychiatric condition which may have been contributing to the behavioral challenges, John did not have a psychiatric diagnosis at the time of the referral for behavioral consultation. He had only a past diagnosis of an adjustment disorder with depressed mood. However, with the symptoms of increased sleep (particularly after the departure of his mother after visits), his increased appetite, his lack of interest in activities, social withdrawal, and his increased irritability (which may have contributed to his aggression), a diagnosis of depression was being considered. Although John had never had a diagnosis of posttraumatic stress disorder, if the behavioral challenges are viewed through the lens of a trauma informed perspective, John had multiple experiences that could have been traumatic for him and created trauma-based responses (i.e., a subthreshold PTSD, if not PTSD). They include the following: neglect and abandonment by his mother growing up; a sense of abandonment that could have been reactivated with her intermittent visits, since she would quickly come and go without consistency or predictability to her visits; change of residences; possible past physical abuse by staff and/or other clients; physical abuse by other clients in his current residence; heart surgery; police intervention that he may not have fully understood; and several psychiatric hospitalizations.

If John's behaviors and symptoms are examined against the specific criteria for posttraumatic stress disorder, he had been exposed to physical abuse or neglect, as well as possible indirect exposure (i.e., watching others in his previous group home being abused and neglected). These criteria (Criterion A – the stressor) would meet the first criteria for the diagnosis of PTSD. Also, his other experiences could have also been traumatic for him even though they don't specifically meet the strict event criteria for PTSD. For example, having to move out of his family home, having to leave his brother's home, living with an aggressive peer, being taken away by police and being psychiatrically hospitalized, undergoing heart surgery as a young child, etc., can all be traumatic experiences.

With regard to Criterion B for PTSD which involves the presence of intrusive symptoms (with one symptom being required for the diagnosis), an argument could be made that his aggressive behavior and his strong reactions to staff approaching him at times could have been "marked physiological reaction after exposure to trauma-related stimuli." He may also have been experiencing some flashbacks of previous abuse and neglect by staff in his other group home which could have been triggering some of his assaults which staff sometimes described as coming "out of the blue."

There were also the instances in which John would show new people his scars. Perhaps John did this because he was afraid and wanted to know that no one will hurt him the way people have hurt him before. Perhaps he showed them because meeting new people triggered fears in him and memories of past abuse. Showing his scars to people he was just meeting may have been his way of communicating his concerns and fears. Once he became familiar with new staff or new people, he ceased displaying his scars. He may have been more likely to be aggressive with new staff because he was scared and unaware of their intentions, given the abuse that may have happened to him in the past. Using these thoughts as working hypotheses, it would become important for anyone supporting him to establish a rapport in order to help him develop a sense of trust and safety.

Criterion C for PTSD involves avoidance reactions in which the individual tries to avoid any situations that may remind him of the trauma. John wanted to avoid medical appointments, and he didn't want to leave the house. However, depression can also result in withdrawal and resistance. Therefore, it is important to remember to consider possible co-morbid or co-occurring conditions. He was also becoming more withdrawn socially, and he didn't want to participate in some of the social events scheduled for the residents in the home.

Criterion D involves negative alterations in someone's thoughts and mood (with two symptoms being required for the diagnosis). One of the criteria in this category includes "markedly diminished interest in significant activities" and "persistent negative trauma-related emotions" which may include anger or fear. John was showing a decrease in his interest to participate in activities and strong emotional reactions at time which were out of proportion to what was actually occurring in the environment or with what was being asked of him.

With regard to Criterion E which includes alterations in arousal and reactivity (with two symptoms being required), John was exhibiting an exaggerated startle response when approached at times. However, it is important to ensure that this is not reflective of a sensory deficit such as a hearing loss. His irritability and aggressive behavior, combined with his exaggerated startle response, may have been reflective of PTSD or at least part of subclinical PTSD presentation.

The diagnosis of PTSD also requires a duration criteria of longer than a month which was the case in John's situation (Criterion F). It also includes Criterion G which specifics that there is "significant symptom-related distress or functional impairment" present which there was in John's case. Criterion H is an exclusionary criterion that states PTSD is not diagnosed if the disturbance is due to substance use, physical illness, or due to a medication side effect. In this particular case, there may have been some medical contributors, but they were not able to be adequately assessed. Since individuals with Down syndrome have a high incidence of sleep apnea such as 50-100% (National Down Syndrome Society.www.ndss.org), excessive fatigue brought on by sleep apnea can contribute to irritability which can lead to aggression and withdrawal due to fatigue. However, it was felt John would not have been cooperative with a sleep study, so his physician did not want to order a sleep study. Therefore, it is possible that there was some medical contributor to John's behavioral presentation given the fact he also had more sleep disruptions when he was having a urinary tract infection.

Interventions

If we operate from the premise that some of John's reactions are both trauma-based and the result of a co-occurring depression, then the interventions need to address these conditions and any possible medical contributors. A treatment plan was devised for John that included the use of some of the Principles of trauma-informed careprinciples of trauma-informed care and some trauma-specific interventions. A trauma- informed approach includes an emphasis on safety (both physical and psychological), trustworthiness, transparency, a strengthening of choice, and the promoting of recovery by building on strengths. The following were some of the interventions which were introduced:

- In order to remove any potential future trauma triggers, the client who assaulted him was given a discharge notice, since it was also felt that he needed a higher level of care. It was hoped that this would have increased John's sense of safety in the home. With a history of probable physical abuse, it would be difficult for John to heal from those memories while still living in an unpre-

dictable situation. No other residents in the home were physically assaultive.
- Since John could not specifically articulate the reasons for lifting his shirt and pointing to his scars, we were left to speculate about the function of this behavior. Several theories were considered: it may have been his way of showing new people how others have hurt him in the past; it may have been his way of also communicating that perhaps he felt unsafe in the presence of new people because he would only do it upon meeting new people; it was also possible that the reasons for him lifting his shirt at this point in time were different than his reasons for engaging in the behavior initially. Sometimes the reasons for a behavior occurring change over time. For example, although he may have displayed his scars to show his distress, it may have changed into an attention-seeking behavior once he realized the attention the action received. Sometimes the reasons that initially cause a behavior to occur may not be the reasons that later maintain the behavior's repeated occurrences. Without knowing for certain (and only being able to hypothesize), a more trauma-focused approach was adopted. New people entering the house were introduced to John by staff members he trusted to help promote a sense of safety for him.
- As John's day was largely unstructured, a visual schedule was introduced. Predictability and control are important dynamics for people with trauma histories. John had stopped attending a day program after he began refusing to leave the house. The visual schedule brought predictability to his day and assured him that he was going to get his needs met. The schedule included pictures of some of his favorite foods. He knew when he was going to eat and what he was going to eat. Choices were also incorporated into the schedule. This also helped to lessen his anxiety because it made his day more predictable.
- Although his mother may have had the best of intentions, the unscheduled visits were difficult for him. Consequently, it was important to talk with her in order to facilitate future visits that could be scheduled in ways that would benefit John. The end of their visits may have been reactivating feelings of abandonment or sadness in him that he didn't know how to manage. He obviously loved his mother, and his affect brightened considerably when he saw her. The administrator for the home explained to both his mother and brother that the best way to support John would be to schedule the visits ahead of time and display them on a calendar (provided his family could commit to the schedule). The administrator also stressed the importance of not setting John up to be disappointed. If it was too difficult for her to commit to a specific date and time in advance, she could call the staff as she was leaving her home so that they could prepare him. Finally, since her leaving was difficult for him after the visits, staff arranged for John to be able to have access to some of his favorite activities afterwards. This allowed him an opportunity to have something to look forward to in an effort to help lessen any sadness and any sense of abandonment. The activities were scheduled with some of his favorite staff members and included food-related outings in which he was able to get some of his favorite foods. Several staff would take him to a drive-through fast food restaurant if he was not showing signs of agitation. In addition, arrangements

were made to change the location of the visit that would allow staff and his family quicker access to leave if John became agitated. They would meet out in the backyard or in a nearby park.
- With scars on his chest and a history of heart surgery, this may have caused painful or fearful memories surrounding doctors' visits. Therefore, changes were instituted regarding appointments. Appointments were scheduled when John could be accompanied by several staff members he trusted, and procedures and the purpose of the visits were explained to him through a variety of methods including gestures, pictures, and modeling. A desensitization procedure was used that involved staff taking him for some of his favorite foods and then driving by the doctor's office. Gradually, this was extended into a walk through the building and then a quick meeting of the office staff. These short visits always ended with a positive association (e.g., a reward of either access to a favorite item or a favorite activity, etc.). In addition, staff also did some role modeling for him. For example, if they were going to take his vitals, the staff had theirs taken so that he could see no harm would come to him.
- At the time of this consultant's observations, John's placement was relatively new and he was still adjusting. Given his experience with staff in his previous group home, he needed time to trust the staff and ensure they were not going to hurt him and that his needs were going to be met. Staff was instructed to approach him slowly and to not startle him. They were also advised to be mindful of physical proximity and to not intrude on his personal space so that he would not feel threatened. They were to avoid any confrontational posturing or any posturing that could be misconstrued as threatening or invasive to him.
- A safe area was created for John in the home where he could be by himself and watch some of his favorite videos. This allowed him time away from the other residents should they have any outbursts so that he could relax and feel safe in that space.
- His psychiatrist was consulted and a provisional diagnosis of PTSD was given. He was also exhibiting some symptoms of depression. Consequently, an antidepressant was prescribed. The antidepressant that was prescribed was also one commonly used to treat PTSD.
- Since John was still undergoing further evaluations to determine the cause of his intermittent enuresis, staff was instructed to contact his physician when John had incidents of bedwetting. His physician could then determine if a urinalysis was necessary in order to rule out a urinary tract infection to ensure that any infections were identified and treated early.
- Interventions included strategies to address his depression such as gradually increasing his activity level, since depression can lead to lethargy and lethargy fuels depression. Also, scheduling some physical activity is also a helpful intervention for addressing depression. Gradually, the staff introduced some activities that John used to find pleasurable. For example, they had him going for short walks with one of his favorite staff followed by a favorite activity (e.g., watching a favorite video or quick van ride to a local fast food drive-thru). They also used his visual schedule that indicated that after he participated

in a short walk he could have access to some rewarding items or activities. Eventually, this was expanded to include his participation in other activities. John became very fond of his visual schedule and would check it various times throughout the day. Because a medical evaluation to rule out of sleep apnea was not able to be completed (which could have continued to cause daytime fatigue and even some signs of depression), John's activities were scheduled later in the day so as to avoid any early morning fatigue. With the introduction of these interventions, John's behaviors and mood improved and his aggression decreased. He was more interactive with staff and cooperative with going to doctors' appointments, and John's residential placement was no longer in jeopardy.

As John's story illustrates, trauma creates a complex puzzle for clinicians to address and many different variables have to be considered. These variables, which can influence behavior, often require a close examination of developmental, medical, and psychological issues.

Michael's Story

Michael was an 18-year-old male who lived in a group home. He was diagnosed with a mild intellectual disability, autism spectrum disorder, and schizoaffective disorder, bipolar type. As Michael was verbal, he could make his needs and wants known, and he was also able to communicate to the staff if he was in any pain or physical discomfort.

Michael had been living at home until his parents could no longer manage his aggressive behavior and his incidents of property destruction. He was aggressive towards both his parents and towards an older sister who was also diagnosed with autism and an intellectual disability in the severe range. His first out-of-home placement occurred when he was 16 years of age when he was admitted to a group home for adolescents. His aggressive behavior became more difficult to manage after his admission, and he was admitted to a psychiatric hospital four times within an eight month period. His hospitalizations varied in length from several days to several weeks. Upon discharge, he returned to the group home until his fourth admission to the psychiatric facility at which time the group home administrator issued a discharge notice. He did not want to accept Michael back to the facility. Consequently, Michael remained at the psychiatric facility for months before being accepted for admission by another group home. While at the hospital, Michael underwent several psychotropic medication changes until his behaviors stabilized. However, the first several weeks of his last hospitalization were difficult. He had been physically aggressive towards the staff. The staff reported that they intervened "quickly and firmly," and he was placed in several physical restraints. The staff felt he was "testing the limits," and they felt it was important that they responded to incidents firmly and consistently. After several restraints and several changes in his psychotropic medications, Michael ceased being aggressive towards the staff. He remained largely to himself at the hospital occasionally asking the staff if he was safe. His family did not visit him while he was residing on the inpatient unit. Michael was described by staff at the hospital as a "loner" who remained rather unmotivated to participate in the unit's activities. However, he was no longer aggressive towards the staff on the unit, and he had not been engaging in property destruction. Consequently, his treatment team at the hospital felt he was ready for discharge, and he was admitted to a new group home. Shortly after being accepted into his new group home he would repeatedly ask if the staff were mean and strict. The staff would respond by saying they were not mean but there were "rules" that needed to be followed.

Michael had been residing in the group approximately one week before his family announced they were going to visit him. His father and mother wanted to see him and told Michael that they would be visiting in two days. One day prior to the visit, he had difficulty sleeping, and he remained highly agitated. He slept only two hours the night before his family was scheduled to come to the home. He was pacing, his speech was more rapid than normal, and he was more talkative than usual. His family came to visit, and the visit went well. He was calm during the visit, and he appeared to enjoy himself. However, within 24 hours after their visit he became agitated and started engaging in acts of property destruction. These included tearing pictures off his wall and ripping some of the items in his room. He then ran to the refrigerator and began eating ice cream, refusing to comply with staff's directions. Michael kept repeating, "Staff are strict," and that he wanted to go home. Later, Michael had difficulty sleeping, and he began to exhibit inappropriate sexual behavior such as trying to masturbate in common areas of the house. He woke early the next morning (after sleeping for only a few hours), and he insisted on calling his family. Since it was 6:00 in the morning, the staff tried to redirect him and inform him that it was too early to call. He responded by threatening to hit the staff member.

Throughout the next 24 hours he engaged in significant property destruction in the home, and he continued to threaten to hit staff. The police were eventually called as the staff was unable to calm him down. Just prior to these events occurring, and just prior to Michael's family visiting, a new resident had been recently admitted to the home who had a very involved family. His family members visited him often. Michael quickly became friends with this new resident, but he would become increasingly agitated and sad whenever his new friend spoke about upcoming visits with his family.

The Analysis

Step 1: Identify the Challenging Behaviors

Michael had a history of property destruction and aggressive behavior prior to his first out-of-home placement. These behaviors prompted his placement, and his behaviors were severe enough at times that he required psychiatric hospitalization. Although his behaviors usually stabilized after being admitted to a psychiatric facility, his progress did not maintain. Just prior to his parents' recent visit, he started to have difficulty sleeping, and he was agitated. In the two days following their visit, he engaged in severe property destruction costing several thousands of dollars to repair. He also started exhibiting sexually inappropriate behavior of trying to masturbate in front of others in the home.

When Michael's challenging behaviors were examined using the *what, where, when,* and *with whom* components of a functional analysis, it was discovered that none of these behaviors were new. These had occurred while he was living at home and in the prior group home. Some of the behaviors (i.e., aggression and property destruction) had also occurred initially after each psychiatric hospitalization but calmed down soon after the hospital admission. Michael's father stated that Michael would occasionally engage in property destruction at home when he was denied something he wanted such as a particular food or activity. Occasionally, he would find Michael masturbating in the living room, and he would quickly tell him to stop. Michael would intermittently experience periods of difficulty sleeping when he would be up most of the night. These periods would be followed by increased sexual activity (frequent episodes of masturbating). These behaviors continued while he was in the first group home but decreased for a period of time with the introduction of psychotropic medications (e.g., antipsychotic medications and a mood stabilizer). However, records from the previous group home noted increases in both his incidents of property destruction and aggression after his parents would visit, and it would take him several days to calm down and have his behaviors return to baseline. Staff at that facility had also reported hearing him cry on occasions while he was taking a shower just prior to their visits and following their visits.

Step 2: Identify the Type and Cause of the Developmental Disability

Michael was diagnosed with autism spectrum disorder and an intellectual disability in the mild range. The cause of either the intellectual disability or the autism was unknown. There was no reference to any genetic syndrome in his records that may have been responsible for the cause of the disabilities in both him and his sister. There was no other family history of any developmental disabilities or psychiatric disorders. However, there are certain behaviors that are commonly exhibited by individuals with autism. For example, they often rigidly adhere to routines which may be a way for them to reduce uncertainty in their environment and any anxiety they may be experiencing. Individuals with autism may also experience greater levels of anxiety, in general, which may increase during periods of change and transition. They may also have specific sensory sensitivities or sensory needs. Behavioral dysregulation can occur if an individual with autism experiences too little sensory input or too much sensory input along different sensory channels.

Step 3: Developmental History/ACEs– Adverse Childhood Experiences

While Michael lived at home not only were his developmental milestones delayed but his family also had to support his sister who had numerous behavioral challenges. While attending school as a child, he also exhibited aggressive behaviors, and he was enrolled in classes with other individuals who had severe behavioral challenges and some of those challenges also included sexual acting out behaviors. Consequently, Michael was able to observe and possibly imitate some behavioral challenges exhibited by his peers.

Because of his escalating behaviors at home, he was forced to leave his family and move into a group home with other peers who had equally, if not more, challenging behaviors. However, he was aware that his sister remained at home. His family's visits were infrequent due to the stress of caring for his disabled sister and the behavioral challenges they were encountering with her. This led to inconsistent visits. There was also a CPS report in his record that referenced allegations of physical abuse by his father. However, the events were never substantiated.

Step 4: Past and Present Psychiatric Diagnoses

In addition to the diagnoses of autism spectrum disorder and a mild intellectual disability, Michael was also diagnosed with schizoaffective disorder, bipolar type. It is unknown from the record when this diagnosis was actually given. This disorder is characterized by symptoms of schizophrenia such as hallucinations or delusions which coexist with symptoms of a mood disorder. There are two forms of the disorder which include either a depressive type or a bipolar type. With the bipolar form an individual will exhibit behaviors which are manic or hypomanic and can include periods of agitation, decreased sleep, and sexualized or impulsive behavior. No other psychiatric diagnoses had been given or noted in Michael's records. There was no official diagnosis of posttraumatic stress disorder even though there were several events that could have been traumatic for him such as having to leave his family home, having to be psychiatrically hospitalized and restrained, intermittent contact with his family, childhood experiences of being around peers with significant behavioral challenges, alleged physical abuse by caretakers, etc. His frequent inquiries about whether or not he was safe and if the staff were going to be strict, along with his incidents of anger outbursts, sleep disturbances, hyperarousal, etc., led to a consideration that some of his behaviors may be reflective of either PTSD (or a subthreshold form of it).

Step 5: Psychotropic Medications

Over several years Michael had undergone numerous changes in his psychotropic medication regimen. He had been prescribed various antipsychotic medications and PRNs for antianxiety medications, as well as an addition of an antidepressant in the past seven months. After his most recent periods of agitation and sexualized behaviors in the home, the psychiatrist introduced a mood stabilizer, lithium. After the introduction of this medication, in addition to the antipsychotic medication he was receiving, as well as an antidepressant medication, Michael's behaviors improved and began to stabilize. However, he began to again manifest some sexualized behaviors and sleep disturbances just prior to his last visit with his parents. His lithium level was low so the dosage was increased. He was also given a medication which could be given on a PRN basis to help him manage his anxiety.

Step 6: Medical Conditions Past and Present

Michael was in good general health with no major health conditions identified other than that he was slightly overweight.

Step 7: Placement History

Michael had his first out-of-home placement as an adolescent. He was separated from his family of origin. Given his frequent statements in which he asked if staff were going to be strict and if he was safe, it can be hypothesized that either the placement itself, the adjustment to placement, or the interactions he had with staff at his first group home had traumatic underpinnings. It was also very difficult for him to be separated from his family, and he would intermittently discuss his sadness about not seeing them and being with them.

Step 8: A Timeline of Events

If a timeline of his life and events is constructed, Michael has had numerous disruptions in his attachment history. He had to leave his parents' home. He was then admitted to an unfamiliar environment without any extended transitional planning. Consequently, he had to adjust to changes in his environment quickly which can be particularly difficult for someone with autism. He had several psychiatric hospitalizations prior to receiving a discharge notice from the first residence. He was then admitted to a new residence and would frequently inquire if the staff were strict and if it was safe. He would also intermittently express sadness about missing his family. In addition to these events, a new resident came to live in the home who had frequent and extensive family involvement which appeared to be difficult for Michael to watch given that his family was not visiting as frequently.

Step 9: Changes in Baseline Functioning

Just prior to Michael's parents visiting this last time, he began to show increased agitation, an increase in speech as well as the rate of his speech, and a decrease in sleep.

Step 10: Current Environment

Although Michael was developing a new friendship with the new resident in the home, there were distinct drawbacks to that relationship. He got to witness first hand all of the attention and caring that his friend's family provided which made him miss his family more. Watching his friend during family visits served as a trigger for some of his sadness and distress and led to some behavioral incidents.

The Final Analysis

Michael has a history of significant losses. He had to leave his family home and move into a congregate living setting with no choice in the matter, since his behavioral challenges were too difficult for his parents to manage. It was clear that he missed his parents and watching the new resident have frequent visits with his family was difficult for him. Michael had a lot of sadness and anger when his family would visit and then leave. His separation from them was very difficult for him. Prior to the last visit with them he began to show some signs that his psychiatric condition of schizoaffective disorder, bipolar type was becoming worse. He was exhibiting some sexualized behaviors, increased agitation, and difficulty sleeping. However, stress can exacerbate psychiatric symptoms, and visiting his parents and having to say good-bye were stressful situations for him. Further, it was discovered that Michael's lithium level was low and out of therapeutic range. It was this medication that helped stabilize his mood and control some of the symptoms of his bipolar form of schizoaffective disorder. Eventually, the combination of all these elements led to a psychiatric admission.

Interventions

Based on all of these factors that were occurring, the following modifications were made to his treatment plan:
- His parents were contacted to see if they would agree to establish more frequent or regular contact. This has been approached with them before, and they had not been receptive. However, given his last psychiatric hospitalization, his interdisciplinary treatment was going to reach out to them again to try and work collaboratively with them for Michael's benefit.
- The behavioral consultant for the home was going to work with Michael on building an affective vocabulary for him. This would help him to identify his feelings prior to acting on them. If he could be helped to more effectively

identify them before they escalated to the point of him engaging in destructive behavior, staff could encourage him to engage in some self-soothing activities. Continued efforts were being made to help Michael develop a repertoire of activities that were calming to him. With the assistance of an occupational therapist, various sensory activities were also explored to add to his repertoire of calming activities.
- Animal assisted activities were also introduced, since it was discovered that Michael loved dogs. The therapist's dog was brought to the facility, and the interactions were closely supervised and the dog assessed to ensure it had the proper temperament.
- Staff was going to arrange to take Michael out in the community when his peer's family was going to visit. If such efforts were proved to be ineffective, the administrator for the residence agreed to have the peer move to his other residence so that Michael would not be frequently triggered by the visits. However, Michael had been developing a strong friendship with his peer, and the staff did not want to discourage it. Therefore, it was agreed that if the peer did move to the administrator's other facility, arrangements would be made for Michael to still see his friend. Activities they both enjoyed (which did not involve family members) were being planned for them such as going to amusement parks and going for bike rides.
- With the assistance of the behavioral consultant for the home, who was also a licensed mental health professional, Michael received instruction in relaxation strategies. These strategies were being rehearsed with him, and staff was also modeling how to do the diaphragmatic breathing during the training sessions and modified progressive muscle relaxation exercises.
- Whenever Michael asked if he was safe, the staff responded very reassuringly. Staff was also instructed to be attentive to the situations that occurred just prior to Michael asking. This was done in an attempt to remove any possible trauma triggers.
- Staff would review a visual schedule daily with Michael so that he knew what to expect during the day. He also was presented with some choices of activities each day. Physical activities were also included in the schedule so that he had physical outlets to release any of his tension or anxiety.
- Staff received training in the signs and symptoms of his psychiatric disorder from the behavioral consultant/therapist. At the earliest signs of any of the symptoms increasing, the psychiatrist was contacted to see if another blood level of the lithium needed to be drawn.
- Trainings were also provided to the staff on supportive and behavioral approaches to use with someone who has a trauma history.

DAVID'S STORY

This particular case is an interesting case as it illustrates the importance of defining trauma not by our definition or experience but by the experience of the individual exposed to the event. David was 23-years-old, and non-verbal, and he lived at home with his mother and father. He had been diagnosed with autism spectrum disorder and an intellectual disability that was in the upper range of moderate. A behavioral consultation was requested because he was refusing to sleep in his room and would sleep on the floor in the living room. He did not want to sleep on the couch but insisted on sleeping on the hard surface of the floor. He refused all attempts made by his mother to persuade him to sleep in his bedroom. He was also becoming increasingly more resistant to leaving the house, and he did not want to attend his day program. He started occasionally refusing to go a few times a week and finally refused to attend at all. This also coincided with his refusal to leave the house and go out into the community with his mother. When his mother would try to insist he leave the house, he would become aggressive with her. When she would take his blanket and pillow and place them back in his bedroom, he would become agitated and engage in either self-injurious behavior (i.e., hitting himself) or aggressive behavior (i.e., hitting her).

David's mother was becoming increasingly frustrated with her son's refusal to leave the house, and she was beginning to feel like "a prisoner" in her own home. The changes in David's behaviors occurred within the past six months. Prior to that, David had been attending a day program and going out in the community with his parents to shop at local retail stores and eat at various restaurants. Although he refused to leave the house to attend his day program or to go to other places in the community, he would agree to go to his doctors' appointments.

The Analysis

Step 1: Identify the Challenging Behaviors.

David was refusing to attend his day program and to leave the house. He was also becoming physically aggressive if he was prompted to go. David also began sleeping on the floor in the living room, and he refused to sleep in his bedroom. He also began to exhibit self-injurious behavior defined as him hitting or slapping himself on the side of the head. David had a history of exhibiting self-injurious behavior and assaultive behavior more frequently when he became an adolescent, but the frequency and intensity decreased over the past few years. He would only intermittently exhibit these behaviors if he was under stress and didn't want to do something. David's refusal to leave the house and his refusal to sleep in his room were new behaviors. His refusal to sleep in his room preceded his refusal to leave the house by approximately a few weeks.

Step 2: Identify the Type and Cause of the Developmental Disabilities

The etiologies of David's autism and intellectual disability were never identified. The developmental disabilities were never attributed to any type of syndrome.

Step 3: Developmental History/ACEs

Upon reviewing his record and interviewing his parents, no significant early childhood experiences were identified as possible sources of trauma. With regard to his developmental milestones, David only spoke a few words as a child and as an adult he become non-verbal. He would use only a few signs to indicate "yes" or "no."

Step 4: Past and Present Psychiatric Diagnoses

David was diagnosed with autism spectrum disorder and an intellectual disability in the moderate range. He did not have a psychiatric diagnosis. However, his mother reported a family history of anxiety on her side of the family. Both her and her mother suffered from severe anxiety which included generalized anxiety and panic attacks which were being treated with antianxiety medications. Her husband also suffered from depression and was being prescribed an antidepressant. David's mother wondered if her son was having any anxiety or panic attacks, since hers had been so bad previously that she did not want to leave the house.

Step 5: Psychotropic Medications

David had been taking the antipsychotic medication, Risperdal, for years due to his aggressive and self-injurious behaviors which he began to exhibit as an adolescent.

Step 6: Medical Conditions Past and Present

David was not being treated for any major medical conditions with the exception of occasional signs of nasal congestion. He had no history of any back or neck injuries or any back problems. Although he would refuse to leave the house to go to his day program or out in the community with his mother, he would agree to see a doctor.

Step 7: Placement History

David lived at home with his parents. They were able to manage his behavioral challenges throughout the years, and they did not want to pursue any out-of-home placement. David did not have any history of psychiatric or medical hospitalizations.

Step 8: Timeline of Events

After interviewing his mother, several significant events were identified which could have contributed to his behavioral issues. David had been sleeping in his room, and the family dog would sleep in his bed with him at night. His parents stated that David was very attached to the dog, but unfortunately, the dog died several months ago. David's refusal to sleep in his bed began approximately one week following the death of his pet. However, since the animal died, David recently began to point to pictures of dogs that he would find in magazines arounds the house. Several weeks after his dog died, one of his favorite job coaches left her job to relocate. A new staff member was assigned to work with him. At around the time this occurred, a new driver for the day program was also assigned to pick David up in the morning. When his mother was asked if there were any events that occurred around the time David began refusing to sleep in his room, she stated that their neighbors had hired a contractor to rebuild a section of their deck on their house. David's bedroom was towards the back of the house, but the construction only lasted a few days.

Step 9: Changes in functioning

Not wanting to sleep in his room was a new behavior for David, and his mother reported that David seemed to have more difficulty falling asleep recently. He did not have a history of sleep difficulties or any changes around his bedtime routines prior to his recent desire to sleep in another room. When asked about any other changes in functioning or behavior, she stated that David's appetite seemed to have decreased in the past few weeks. There were changes in his motivation, and he did not want to attend the day program, but spent most of his day just sitting in the living room watching his IPad.

Step 10: Current environment

With regard to his current environment, his mother had reported she was experiencing more stress and anxiety since it was difficult for her to leave the house because of David's behaviors. She felt resentful and "trapped" by her son's behaviors. Admittedly, she said this led to her being a little more irritable and impatient with David. This was combined with her husband having to work more overtime at his job.

The Final Analysis

There are a number of issues which arise as a timeline of events was recreated for David. Obviously, he was attached to his dog and the dog's death was a loss for him. He was also experiencing the loss of a staff member who he had known and worked with for a long time. Around the time of these losses, a new driver was assigned to pick him up and take him to his day program. While these events were occurring, his father was not home as often, and David would often spend time in the early evening with his father watching television. This represented another change or loss for him. With David's diagnosis of autism spectrum disorder, changes and transitions were difficult and anxiety provoking for him. There was also a significant family history of anxiety disorders which may have also increased the probability of David developing one. Although these events may be stressful and not considered to be traumatic by some, they could have been traumatic for David resulting in increased anxiety. Since some people with autism have heightened sensitivities to certain sensory input such as certain sounds, or sights, etc., it is also possible that the sounds emanating from the contractor's work were aversive to him or even traumatic. This could have contributed to his resistance to sleep in his room and his refusal leave the house. However, since David was non-verbal, these were hypotheses that were generated to try and explain the reasons motivating his behaviors. (This is what is also done in a functional analysis. Hypotheses are formed regarding the functions of the behaviors, interventions are introduced, and the hypotheses are tested.)

Interventions

Based on the analysis of all of the possible contributors to his behaviors, the approach that was used involved several interventions, including trauma sensitive interventions and consisted of the following:
- It included trying to help him process the loss of his pet. His parents had taken the dog to the veterinarian, and the dog had been euthanized due to illness. However, David had not been involved in the process, and he did not receive much of an explanation of what happened. Consequently, he may not have fully understood why his dog was not coming back or had a chance to even process his grief. It was recommended that his parents try to explain what happened. Since David likes to use pictures, they could use pictures to try and convey the sequence of events. There were also books about grief due to the loss of animals that they could purchase and read to him (suited to his developmental level), since he had a collection of books in his room which he liked to read. In addition, since he loved animals and his dog may have helped to calm him down or ease anxieties for him, his parents were considering getting another dog for him. However, in the interim, his love of animals was used as motivation to try and motivate him to leave the house. His uncle, who lived nearby, had a very friendly dog. His parents showed him pictures of the dog and asked if he would stop by with the dog. David's affect brightened

when he saw the dog and his uncle invited him to come to visit. This was used as an incentive to schedule short trips to his uncle's house to increase his activity level and promote more social connectedness.
- The construction noises that had occurred may have made it aversive or fearful for him to sleep in his room. Consequently, his parents changed the location of his bedroom and had him help arrange the furniture. Since they found him sleeping with a lot of blankets on top of him, they bought him a sleeping bag initially to put on his bed. He seemed to like the comfort of feeling somewhat enclosed. An occupational therapy consultation was eventually sought and a weighed blanket was recommended.
- After David's behaviors started to improve, his parents asked if one of the staff that he had worked with previously could be assigned to work with him at the day program. The day program administrator agreed, and his parents explained to David that one of his other favorite staff would be working with him. They had her assigned to help with transporting in the morning so that David felt more comfortable getting on the van.
- Once David felt more comfortable going out, another desensitization procedure was used to start taking him to other places in the community. His mother would take him for short visits starting with a ride to a fast food drive-through. These trips were gradually extended to include taking longer routes to get to the fast food restaurants so David could get used to leaving the house again.
- A doctor's appointment was made for him to get a physical. After making an appointment for him, it was discovered he had a very bad sinus infection, and he was treated with antibiotics. Following some of the doctors' appointments, his mother would take him over to his uncle's home to visit with the dog.
- Since David's mother's stress level had been increasing because she was unable to get a break and leave the house, her interactions with her son were becoming more negative. Consequently, additional respite services were added that allowed her to get out of the house and take a break from the stress of being a full-time caretaker.
- Due to a significant family history of anxiety, it was thought that David may be also experiencing some underlying anxiety. Where there is anxiety, there may also be depression. Consequently, a psychiatric consultation was scheduled, and he was prescribed an antianxiety medication on a PRN basis which his mother stated seemed to help him and he appeared much calmer and more cooperative.

CASE REFLECTIONS

It becomes apparent after reviewing these individuals' stories that getting to know the individuals and the various events or factors that can influence their behaviors can be a time-consuming process. It requires not only a commitment of time but also a commitment to try and understand what their lives have been like. However, the more you learn about the person, the easier it becomes to try and understand their behavioral challenges. If a person is verbal, the process is easier provided the individual is able to identify and articulate the issues and their feelings about the situations. It can certainly be more challenging and require more detective work when the individual is non-verbal.

Uncovering traumas, either small or large events or an accumulation of stressful events, which may be causing or contributing to the behavioral challenges, is an important part of understanding someone's life story. Interventions to address those traumas or stress-related events may need to include a multipronged strategy. Such a strategy may involve a variety of approaches, some specifically geared towards addressing trauma, some interventions geared towards promoting resiliency, some towards addressing medical issues and addressing any co-occurring psychiatric conditions, and some towards addressing learned behaviors. A multipronged treatment approach is often needed due to the complexity of issues frequently faced by individuals with developmental disabilities.

Often individuals with trauma histories can face a variety of issues that are often not fully appreciated by others and present a complexity of challenges. They may have experienced many disruptions in their lives due to changes in caretakers, changes in residences, changes in health status, etc. Consequently, it is not unusual for some of them, particularly with traumatic backgrounds, to also have severe behavioral reputations. Their behavioral challenges continue to increase as more disruptions are introduced such as placement changes, psychiatric hospitalizations, and numerous medication changes. These changes continue and eventually the interventions become increasingly ineffective. A thorough understanding of the path that led to the current situation becomes a more distant reality. However, this type of a life review becomes even more imperative as the behavioral challenges increase and there is a history of ineffective interventions. Although this level of analysis is time consuming, consider the amount of time and money that often is invested without successful results while interventions continue to fail. More importantly, consider the adverse impact such failures have on the individual's quality of life, their family members, and the individual's morale.

Chapter 9

A Summary

When working with individuals who have both intellectual disabilities and experiences which have produced trauma, it is important to be sensitive to how their trauma has impacted their behaviors and relationships with others. The impact of trauma can weave itself into many different aspects of their daily lives. The identification of PTSD and its manifestations and the creation of appropriate interventions and treatments are much needed areas of study among this population. There is a significant lack of systematic research that includes rigorously controlled studies to identify the most effective treatments for PTSD among this population, despite the high prevalence rate of abuse among individuals with developmental disabilities. As clinicians and care providers who support individuals with intellectual disabilities, we are left to extract and extrapolate from the findings of the studies on PTSD conducted among the general population. We have to rely on our own experiences in applying and modifying those findings in the absence of specific studies targeting this population. Consequently, this book is meant to serve as a primer. It is a beginning step in the need to increase awareness and sensitivity in assessing for trauma and supporting individuals who have been exposed to traumatic experiences. It is a particularly important topic to be sensitive to when supporting individuals with ID who have severe behavioral reputations. Often their histories are marked by numerous disruptions in their living situations and in their relationships. Too often the focus is on the modification of their behaviors through a variety of behavior management strategies such as various reward systems, contingency contracting, environmental modifications, and through the use of psychotropic medications. These measures are undertaken without a full appreciation of the variables that have contributed to their behavioral challenges such as the existence of traumatic experiences.

Arguments have been made by some authors in the field of trauma that in order to increase the awareness regarding the prevalence of trauma and its sequelae, care providers, and those working in health care arenas should consider trauma-informed interventions as a form of universal precautions. For example, when individuals are treated in a health care setting and universal precautions are implemented, medical personnel adopt procedures such as the use of gloves when handling bodily fluids and the use of surface disinfectants, etc. The assumption behind the use of universal precautions is that everyone has the potential to carry some infectious process which may be communicable. If this principle is extended to trauma care, then considering traumatic stress as a potential factor influencing present behaviors should be the norm when supporting individuals with intellectual disabilities. Consequently, introducing interventions that promote safety, choice, and control are of primary importance. If the individual has not had a traumatic history, then there is no loss in adopting this assumption. After all, what is the harm in still helping individuals to feel safe and to feel as though they have some choice and control in their lives?

An important element in providing trauma-informed care is to ensure that a screening mechanism exists for trauma, and this type of approached is emphasized regardless of the types of services the person is accessing (e.g., outpatient mental health or medical treatment, etc.). Without some form of screening and identification, care systems may fail to meet the needs of the individual potentially rendering treatments ineffective. The absence of these protocols increases the risk that organizations will implement policies and procedures that may unintentionally re-traumatize those they seek to serve. Being aware of trauma-based behaviors and symptoms that may be reflective of PTSD, or even sub-threshold PTSD, in individuals with intellectual disabilities can help to identify the proper supports and services that are needed.

The concept of having trauma-informed or trauma-sensitive service workers, care providers, and clinicians speaks to the unique needs of supporting individuals whose life experiences have impacted their behaviors. Without this sensitivity, there is a risk of inadvertently adding to their distress, as well as creating ineffective care or behavior plans, whose failures become predicated on not factoring in a significant underlying cause of the behavior (i.e., trauma). By not introducing the proper services and supports, their healing can be compromised, or it may not happen at all. In supporting individuals with dual diagnoses and working within the frame work of trauma informed care, it is important to remember the following points:

- Be aware and be sensitive to their life histories. If you support them, get to know them. Know their histories and know where they have been and what they have been through. Try to get some understanding of what it may have been like to "walk in their shoes" but don't evaluate trauma by your own set of standards. There is individual variability in the experience and perception of traumatic events even though some events are universally considered to be traumatic.
- Be particularly sensitive to early childhood experiences of abandonment by biological parents or a history of disruptions in major attachments in their lives.
- Be sensitive to any early adverse childhood experiences (ACEs) the individual may have had since this can have profound and long lasting effects.
- Be sensitive to the experiences of individuals who have lived in congregate settings. Remember, many individuals with intellectual disabilities have lived in a variety of residential settings with peers they didn't know. They may not have had a voice in deciding on the living arrangement. While living in congregate settings, they may have been exposed to the disruptive and sometimes threatening behaviors of their peers, particularly if the home was identified to support individuals with behavioral challenges. Imagine how you would you feel if you had to live with others who yelled, who were unpredictable, who became assaultive or threatened others, who destroyed property, or who generally made the environment feel unsafe.

- Look at the individual's history(s) with their caretakers. Were their care takers or other individuals in their support systems generally concerned with their well-being? Were care takers attentive? Is there a history of physical, emotional, or financial abuse or negligence by anyone who was once in the position of providing care?
- Did care providers establish healthy boundaries? Where the caretakers controlling, or were they so permissive that boundaries were never clearly drawn? These characteristics add to a feeling of uncertainty and a lack of safety. We feel safer when we know what to expect of others and what is expected of us. Boundaries keep us safe on many levels. Consequently, it is important for individuals with ID who are living in adult residential facilities or group homes to be supported by staff who can establish and maintain healthy boundaries. It is also helpful if staff turnover is not high, since consistent and healthy relationships can help the individual to heal. Consistency builds trust, and trust is often a casualty of trauma.
- Remember that helping to reestablish a sense of safety and control is very important for anyone who has undergone trauma. Help create environments that are safe and free from trauma triggers that re-stimulate painful memories or experiences.
- Whenever possible provide choices and more opportunities for choice. This will promote a feeling of having more control. A sense of helplessness and a lack of control can be part and parcel for those who have had traumatic experiences.
- Acknowledge and promote strengths. Remember the factors that facilitate resiliency in the general population, and provide opportunities to develop confidence whenever possible.
- Be respectful in your interactions. Avoid coercive interventions as well as interventions that run the risk of re-traumatizing the individual.
- Remember that there are many different types of trauma but a more finite number of reactions. What may be traumatizing to one individual may not be traumatizing to another. There is a level of individuality in this area which needs to be appreciated. Avoid judging another person's experience and avoid defining an event as traumatic by your own standards. Although it can be agreed that certain events would be considered traumatic by a majority of people, the events may not produce PTSD. Not everyone who has experienced a traumatic event is traumatized. Not everyone who goes through a traumatic event develops PTSD. This is where a host of individual factors come into play in mediating someone's reactions.
- Although someone's symptoms may not meet the criteria for a diagnosis of PTSD, be sensitive to the possibility that the individual may be experiencing subthreshold PTSD (i.e., experiencing some symptoms but not enough to meet the diagnosis).
- It is important to consider the possibility that long standing, challenging behaviors may have their origin in part, or in whole, out of trauma which happened years ago. This can become easily overlooked when considering the length of time the behaviors have been occurring.

- Do not fail to report abuse or neglect. Do not remain silent. Individuals with developmental disabilities can be a vulnerable population for all the reasons previously discussed. Help them have a voice.
- When working within a health care delivery system supporting individuals with intellectual and developmental disabilities, be guided by the Principles of trauma-informed care principles of trauma-informed care which emphasizes the need to promote personal choice, mutuality, and collaboration. If you work within a system that contributes to the re-traumatization of the individual, don't remain silent. Do your best to educate, advocate, and increase awareness so that the system can make needed modifications.
- Remember that in supporting individuals with developmental disabilities who may have experienced trauma, be sensitive to the fact their families or care providers supporting them may also be experiencing such reactions. The stress of prolonged caring for a loved one with a disability may produce traumatic-like responses in caretakers. The stress may also result in families who present with an angry or adversarial approach. Consider that their responses may be born out of prolonged stress, fatigue, and a sense of helplessness and hopelessness. Collaborate. Help empower those families. Most of all, respect what they have been trying to do, the journey they have been on, and the stress they have been under.
- Most importantly, remember that healing is possible, and people can be very resilient. However, it is difficult, if not impossible, to heal in an environment that continually provides trauma triggers. Healing environments which emphasize safety, choice, healthy boundaries, positive experiences, and good social support provide the elements which are critical to healing.

The Future

Within the past several decades, the concept of providing trauma-informed care has been emerging and finding its way into mental health arenas, health care settings, the foster care system, and even in educational areas. However, providing trauma-informed care to individuals with intellectual disabilities is an area that continues to need greater attention. Trauma-informed systems and greater screening and assessment methods are needed for the identification and treatment of PTSD and trauma-based responses among this population. Such an approach will help ensure that service delivery systems are cognizant in identifying trauma and its sequelae. By doing so, these systems can help to mitigate the effects of trauma on individuals with intellectual disabilities and facilitate the healing process.

Historically, the focus has been on addressing behavioral challenges among individuals with developmental disabilities and has included looking at the function of those behaviors. Often the function of the challenging behavior has been identified as serving an attention-seeking, task avoidance function or a release of tension, and it has not often been viewed as a trauma-based reaction. For those individuals with intellectual disabilities who present with severe behavioral challenges, which have been caused or exacerbated by trauma, adopting a trauma-informed approach will not only help to facilitate empathy and understanding in others, but it will provide a better conceptual framework in which to approach these challenges. If the findings from neuroscience are considered, then therapeutic approaches to addressing PTSD in individuals with developmental disabilities should include an emphasis on re-establishing a balanced autonomic nervous system.

Unaddressed trauma can increase the risk of psychological issues, physical disorders, and substance abuse as well as other addictive behaviors. Individuals with intellectual disabilities and trauma histories have been known to all service delivery systems such as the juvenile and correctional system, the foster care system, and the mental health system. Their needs are not just isolated to the developmental disabilities system. It is important to ensure that all service sectors are trauma-sensitive so that the very services provided by these organizations are not trauma-inducing themselves.

Trauma-informed care should occur not only at the service level but also at the organizational level. It acknowledges the need to not only understand the clientele it serves, but it also focuses on promoting provider and staff well-being. Providing trauma-informed care will help to improve the quality of the lives of individuals with developmental disabilities and even the lives of those who support them. Providing thoughtful, relevant care to the often misunderstood population of individuals with intellectual disabilities is the best way to ensure each individual is given the tools needed to thrive and not just survive.

References

Adams. E. (2010). Healing invisible wounds: Why investing in trauma-informed care for children makes sense. *Justice Policy Institute, July,* 1-15.

Adams, R.E., Boscarino, J.A., & Galea, S. (2006). Alcohol use, mental health status and psychological well-being two years after the World Trade Center attacks in New York City. *The American Journal of Drug and Alcohol Abuse, 32,* 203-224.

Alexander, C.N., Swanson, G.C., Rainforth, M.V., Carlisle, T.W., Todd, C.C., & Oates, R.M., Jr. (1993). Effects of the transcendental meditation program on stress reduction, health, and employee development: A prospective study in two occupational settings. *Anxiety, Stress and Coping: An International Journal, 6*(3), 245-262.

Allen, K.D., & Kupzyk, S. (2016). Compliance with medical routines. In J.K.Luiselli (Ed.), *Behavioral health promotion and intervention in intellectual and developmental disabilities* (pp. 21-42). Switzerland: Springer International.

American Psychiatric Association. (1952). *Diagnostic and statistical manual of mental disorders* (1st ed.). Washington, DC: Author.

American Psychiatric Association. (1968). *Diagnostic and statistical manual of mental disorders* (2nd ed.). Washington, DC: Author.

American Psychiatric Association. (1980). *Diagnostic and statistical manual of mental disorders* (3rd ed.). Washington, DC: Author.

American Psychiatric Association. (1987). *Diagnostic and statistical manual of mental disorders* (3rd ed. revised). Washington, DC: American Psychiatric Association.

American Psychiatric Association. (1994). *Diagnostic and statistical manual of mental disorders* (4th ed.). Washington, DC: Author.

American Psychiatric Association. (2000). *Diagnostic and statistical manual of mental disorders* (4th ed. text revision).Washington. DC: Author.

American Psychiatric Association. (2013). *Diagnostic and statistical manual of mental disorders* (5th ed.). Washington, DC: Author.

Aupperle, R.L., Melrose, A.J., Stein, M.B., & Paulus, M.P. (2012). Executive function and PTSD: Disengaging from trauma. *Neuropharmacology, 62*(20), 686-694.

Babbel, S. (2011). Medical trauma: When a procedure goes wrong. *Psychology Today.* Retrieved from https://www.psychologytoday.com/blog.somatic-psychology/201110/medical-trauma-when-procedure-goes wrong.

Baladerian, N.J. (2013). *Trauma and people with intellectual or developmental disabilities: Recognizing signs of abuse and providing effective symptom relief.* Presentation West Virginia Integrated Behavioral Health Conference.

Baranowsky, A.B., & Gentry, J.E. (2014). *Trauma practice: Tools for stabilization and recovery.* Boston, MA: Hogrefe.

Barnes, V.A., Schneider, R., Alexander, C., & Staggers, F. (1997). Stress, stress reduction, and hypertension in African Americans. *Journal of the National Medical Association, 89,* 464-476.

Barnes V.A., Rigg, J.L., & Williams, J.J. (2013). Clinical case series; treatment of PTSD with Transcendental Meditation in active duty military personnel. *Military Medicine, 178*(7), 836-840.

Barol, B.J., & Seubert, A. (2010). Stepping stones: EMDR treatment of individuals with intellectual and developmental disabilities and challenging behavior. *Journal of EMDR Practice and Research, 4*(4), 156-169.

Barrowcliff, A. (2008). Cognitive-behavioral therapy for command hallucinations and intellectual disability: A case study. *Journal of Applied Research in Intellectual Disability, 21*(3), 236-245.

Barrowcliff, A.L., & Evans, G.A. (2015). EMDR treatment for PTSD and intellectual disability: A case study. *Advances in Mental Health and Intellectual Disabilities, 9*(2), 90-98.

Bar-Shalita, T., & Cermak, S.A. (2016). Atypical sensory modulation and psychological distress in the general population. *American Journal of Occupational Therapy, 70*(4).

Beetz, A., Uvnas-Moberg, K., Julius, H., & Kotrschal, K. (2012). Psychosocial and psychophysiological effects of human-animal interactions: The possible role of oxytocin. *Frontiers in Psychology, 3*, 234.

Benson, B.A., & Fuchs, C. (1999). Anger-arousing situations and coping responses of aggressive adults with intellectual disability. *Journal of Intellectual and Developmental Disability, 24*(3), 207-214.

Bergmann, V. (2008). The neurobiology of EMDR. Exploring the thalamus and neural integration. *Journal of EMDR Practice and Research, 2*, 300-314.

Black, D., & Rosenthal, N. (2015). Transcendental medication for autism spectrum disorders? A perspective. *Cogent Psychology, 2*, 1-5.

Blair, C., & Diamond, A. (2008). Biological processes in prevention and intervention: The promotion of self-regulation as a means of preventing school failure. *Development and Psychopathology, 20*, 899-911.

Blevins, C.A., Weathers, F.W., Davis, M.T., Witte, T.K., & Domino, J.L. (2015). The Posttraumatic Stress Disorder Checklist for DSM-5 (PCL-5): Development and initial psychometric evaluation. *Journal of Traumatic Stress, 28*, 489-498.

Boscarino, J.A., (1997). Diseases among men 20 years after exposure to severe stress: Implications for clinical research and medical care. *Psychosomatic Medicine, 59*(6), 605-614.

Bosson J., Reuther, E., & Cohen, A. (2011). The comorbidity of psychotic symptoms and post-traumatic stress disorder: Evidence of a specifier in DSM-5. *Clinical Schizophrenia and Related Psychosis, 5*(3), 147-154.

Brady, K.T., Killeen, T.K., Brewerton, T., & Lucerini, S. (2000). Co-morbidity of psychiatric disorders and posttraumatic stress disorder. *Journal of Clinical Psychiatry, 61*(7), 22-32.

Brady, K., Pearlstein, T., Asnis, G.M., Baker, D., Rothbaum, B., Sikes, C.R., & Farfel, G.M. (2000). Efficacy and safety of Sertraline treatment of posttraumatic stress disorder: A randomized controlled trial. *Journal of the American Medical Association, 28*, 1837-1844.

Breslau, N., Chilcoat, H.D., Kessler, R.C., Peterson, E.L., & Lucia, V.C. (1999). Vulnerability to assaultive violence: Further specification of the sex difference in post-traumatic stress disorder. *Psychological Medicine, 29*(4), 813-821.

Breslau, N., Kessler, R.C., Chilcoat, H.D., Schultz, L.R., Davis, G.C., & Andreski, P. (1998). Trauma and posttraumatic stress disorder in the community: The 1996 Detroit area survey of trauma. *Archives of General Psychiatry, 156*, 360-366.

Breslau, N., Lucia, V.C., & Alvarado, G.F. (2006). Intelligence and other predisposing factors in exposure to trauma and posttraumatic stress disorder. *Archives of General Psychiatry, 11,* 1238-45.

Breslau, N., Wilcox, H., Storr, C., Lucia, V., & Anthony, J.C. (2004). Trauma exposure and posttraumatic stress disorder: A study of youth in urban America. *Journal Urban Health. 81*(4), 530-544.

Briere, J. (2005). *Trauma Symptom Checklist for young children: Professional manual.* Odessa, Florida: Psychological Assessment Resources, Inc.

Brickell, C., & Munir, K. (2008). Grief and its complications in individuals with intellectual disability. *Harvard Review of Psychiatry, 16*(1), 1-12.

Brown, J.F., Brown, M.Z., & Dibiasio, P. (2013). Treating individuals with intellectual disabilities and challenging behaviors with adapted dialectical behavior therapy. *Journal of Mental Health Research Intellectual Disabilities, 6*(4), 280-303.

Brown, C., & Dunn, W. (2002). *Adolescent/adult sensory profile manual.* San Antonio, TX: Psychological Corporation.

Calhoun, P.S., Wiley, M., Dennis, M.F., & Beckham, J.C. (2009). Self-reported health and physician diagnosed illnesses in women with posttraumatic stress disorder and major depressive disorder. *Journal of Traumatic Stress, 22*(2), 122-130.

Carr, R.B. (2011). Combat and human existence: Towards an intersubjective approach to combat-related PTSD. *Psychoanalytic Psychology, 28* (4), 471-496.

Center for Disease Control and Kaiser Permanente (1998). Relationship of childhood abuse and household dysfunction to many of the leading causes of death in adults. *American Journal of Preventative Medicine, 14,* 245-258.

Champagne, T. (2003). Creating nurturing and healing environments for enhancing a culture of care. *Occupational Therapy Advance, 19* (19), 50.

Chapman, R.A., Shedlack, K.J., & France, J. (2006). Stop-think-relax: An adapted self-control training strategy for individuals with mental retardation and coexisting psychiatric illness. *Cognitive and Behavioral Practice, 13*(3), 205-214.

Chen, M.Y., Wang, E.K., & Jeng, YJ. (2006). Adequate sleep among adolescents is positively associated with health status and health-related behaviors. *BMC Public Health, 8*(6), 59.

Cloud, H. & Townsend (1995). *Boundaries.* Grand Rapids, Michigan: Zondervan.

Coentre, R., & Power, P. (2011). A diagnostic dilemma between psychosis and post-traumatic stress disorder: A case report and review of the literature. *Journal of Medical Case Reports, 5,* 97.

Cole, P.M., Michel, M.K., & Teti, L.O. (1994). The developmental of emotional regulation and dysregulation: A clinical perspective. *Monographs of the Society for Research in Child Development, 59*(2-3), 73-102.

Cooper, J.L. (2007). Facts about trauma for policy makers: Children's Mental Health. National Center for Children in Poverty. New York, NY. Retrieved March 10, 2017 from www.ncpp.org

Cooper, S.A., Smiley, E., Morrison, J. Williamson, A., & Allan, L. (2007). Mental ill-health in adults with intellectual disabilities: prevalence and associated factors. *British Journal of Psychiatry, 190,* 27-35.

Corray, S.E., & Bakala, A. (2005). Anxiety disorders in people with learning disabilities. *Advances in Psychiatric Treatment, 11,* 355-361.

Cottis, T. (Ed.) (2008). *Intellectual disability, trauma and psychotherapy*. London: Routledge.

Covey, S., (1989). *The 7 habits of highly effective people*. New York, New York: Free Press.

Cozolino, L. (2010). *The neuroscience of psychotherapy: Healing the social brain* (2nd ed.). New York, NY: Norton.

Cukor, J., Spitalnick, J., Difede, J., Rizzo, A, & Rothbaum, B.O. (2009). Emerging treatments for PTSD. *Clinical Psychology Review, 29*(8), 715-726.

Cukor, J., Wyka, K., Jayasinghe, N., & Difede. J.A. (2010). The nature and course of subthreshold PTSD. *Journal of Anxiety Disorders, 24*(8), 918-923.

Daniel, B. (2007). The concept of resilience: messages for residential child care. In: Kendrick. (Ed.), *Residential child care: Prospects and challenges*. Research Highlights in Social Work Series, (pp. 60-75). London: Jessica Kingsley.

De Kloet, E.R., Karst, H., & Joels, M. (2008). Corticosteroid hormones in the central response: Quick-and-slow. *Frontiers in Neuroendocrinology, 29*, 268-272.

Doidge, N. (2015). *The brain's way of healing*. New York, New York: Viking Press.

Durand, V.M., & Barlow, D.H. (2006). Anxiety disorders. M. Taflinger (Ed.), *Essentials of abnormal psychology* (pp. 155-161). Belmont, CA: Thomas Wardsworth.

Duric, N.S., Assmus, J., Gundersen, D., & Elgen, I.B. (2012). Neurofeedback for the treatment of children and adolescents with ADHD: A randomized and controlled clinical trial using parental reports. *BMC Psychiatry 12*, 107.

Dykstra, E., & Charlton, M. (2003). Dialectical behavior therapy skills training: Adapted for special population. Unpublished manuscript, Aurora Mental Health Center, Intercept Center 11023 E 5th Avenue, Aurora, CO 80010.

Emerson, P. (1977). Covert grief reaction in mentally retarded clients. *Mental Retardation, 15*(6), 46-47.

Eppley, K.R., & Abrams, A.L. (1989). Differential effects of relaxation techniques on trait anxiety: A meta-analysis. *Journal of Clinical Psychology, 45*, 957-974.

Epsie, C., & Mindham, J. (2003). Glasgow Anxiety Scale for people with an Intellectual Disability (GAS-ID): Developmental and psychometric properties of a new measure for use with people with mild intellectual disability. *Journal of Intellectual Disability Research, 47*, 22-30.

Esbensen, A.J., & Benson, B.A. (2006). A prospective analysis of life events, problem behaviors and depression in adults with intellectual disability. *Journal of Intellectual Disability Research, 4*, 248-258.

Eyerman, J. (1981). Transcendental meditation and mental retardation. *Journal of Clinical Psychiatry, 42*, 35-36.

Fabes, R.A., Einsenberg, N., Karbon, M., Troyer, D., & Switzer, G. (1994). The relations of children's emotion regulation to their vicarious emotional responses and comforting behaviors. *Child Development, 65*, 1687-1693.

Fallot. R.D., & Harris, M. (2009). *Creating cultures of trauma-informed care (CCTIC): A self-assessment and planning protocol*. Peoria, IL: Community Connections.

Firth, H., Balogh, R., Berney, T., Bretherton, K., Graham, S., & Whibley, S. (2001). Psychopathology of sexual abuse in young people with intellectual disability. *Journal of Intellectual Disability Research, 45*(3), 244-252.

Fletcher, R.J., Barnhill, J., & Cooper, S. (2016). *Diagnostic manual intellectual disability: A textbook of diagnosis of mental disorders in persons with intellectual disability*. Kingston, NY: NADD Press.

Fletcher, R., Loschen, E., Stavrakaki, C., & First, M. (Eds). (2007). *Diagnostic manual-intellectual disability (DM-ID): A textbook of diagnosis of mental disorders in persons with intellectual disability.* Kingston, NY: NADD Press.

Foa, E.B., Johnson, K.M., Feeny, N.C., & Treadwell, K.R.H. (2001). The Child PTSD Symptom Scale: A preliminary examination of its psychometric properties. *Journal of Clinical Child Psychology, 30,* 376 – 384.

Focht-New, G., Clements, P.T., Barol, B., Faulkner, M.J., & Pekala, K. (2008). Persons with developmental disabilities exposed to interpersonal violence and crime: Strategies and guidance for assessment. *Perspectives in Psychiatric Care, 44*(1), 3-13.

Ford, J. & Honnor, J. (2000). Job satisfaction of community residential staff serving individuals with severe intellectual disabilities. *Journal of Intellectual and Developmental Disability, 25,* 343-62.

Foy, D.W., Sipprelle, R.C., Rueger, D.B., & Carroll, E.M. (1984). Etiology of posttraumatic stress disorder in Vietnam veterans: Analysis of pre-military, military, and combat exposure influences. *Journal of Consulting and Clinical Psychology, 52*(1), 79-87.

Frans, O., Rimmo, P.A., Aberg, L., & Fredrikson, M. (2005). Trauma exposure and post-traumatic stress disorder in the general population. *Acta Psychiatrica Scandinavica, 111*(4), 291-9.

Friedman, M.J. (2000). *Posttraumatic stress disorder: The latest assessment and treatment strategies.* Kansas City, MO: Compact Clinicals.

Gentile, J.P., & Gillig, P.M. (2012). *Psychiatry of intellectual disability: A practical manual.* Hoboken, NJ: Wiley and Sons.

Gilbertson, M.W., Shenton, M.E., Ciszewski, A., Kasai, K., Lasko, N.B., Orr, S.P., Pitman, R.K. (2002). Smaller hippocampal volume predicts pathological vulnerability to psychological trauma. *Nature Neuroscience, 5,* 1242 – 1247.

Gilderthorp, R.C. (2015). Is EMDR an effective treatment for people diagnosed with both intellectual disability and posttraumatic stress disorder? *Journal of Intellectual Disabilities, 19,* (1), 58-68.

Gillis, J.M., Hammond Natof, T., Lockshin, S.B., & Romanczyk, R.G. (2009). Fear of routine physical exams in children with autism spectrum disorders: Prevalence and intervention effectiveness. *Focus on Autism and Other Developmental Disabilities, 24,* 156-168.

Giltaij, H. (2004). Alsof er een stofzuiger door mijn hoofd is gegann. EMDR bij mensen met een visuele en verstandelijke beperking. (EMDR in people with visual and intellectual disabilities.) *Tijdschrift voor Kinder & Jeugdpsychotherapie, 3,* 81-97.

Grandner, M.A., Kripke, D.F., Naidoo, N., & Langer, R.D. (2010). Relationship among dietary nutrients and subjective sleep, objective sleep, and napping in women. *Sleep Medicine, 11*(2),180.

Green, B.L. (1991). Evaluating the effects of disasters. *Psychological Assessment: A Journal of Consulting and Clinical Psychology, 3,* 538-546.

Greenberg, M.T. (2006). Promoting resilience in children and youth: preventative interventions and their interface with neuroscience. *Annals of the New York Academy of Sciences,* 1094, 139-150.

Gustaffson, C., & Sonnander, K. (2004). Occurrences of mental health problems in Swedish samples of adults with intellectual disabilities. *Social Psychiatry and Psychiatric Epidemiology, 39*(6), 448-456.

Hagland, M., Cooper, N., Southwick, S., & Charney, D. (2007). 6 keys to resilience for PTSD and everyday stress. *Current Psychiatry, 6*(4), 23-30.

Hall, M.F. & Hall, S.E. (2013). *When treatment becomes trauma: Defining, preventing, and transforming medical trauma.* Paper based on a program presented at the 2013 American Counseling Association Conference, Cincinnati, Ohio.

Hall, J.C., Jobson, L., & Langdon, P.E. (2014). Measuring symptoms of post-traumatic stress disorder in people with intellectual disabilities: the development and psychometric properties of the Impact of Event Scale-Intellectual Disabilities (IES-IDs). *British Journal of Clinical Psychology, 53*(3), 315 – 332.

Halligan, S.L., & Yehuda, R. (2000). Risk factors for PTSD. *PTSD Research Quarterly, 11*(3), 1050-1835.

Hamblen, J., & Barnett, E. (2009). PTSD in children and adolescents. National Center for PTSD. Retrieved from http://www.ptsd.va.gov/professional/pages.

Harrell, E. (2017). Crime against persons with disabilities 2009 – 2015 – Statistical tables. *Bureau of Justice Statistics.* http://www.bjs.gov/index.cfm?ty=pbdetail&iid=4574.

Harris, M., & Fallot, R. (2001). *Using trauma theory to design service system.* San Francisco, CA: Jossey-Bass.

Hatton, C., & Emerson, E. (2004). The relationship between life events and psychopathology amongst children with intellectual disabilities. *Journal of Applied Research in Intellectual Disabilities, 17,*109-117.

Hebb, D.O. (1949). *Organization of behavior.* New York, NY: Wiley.

Heiger, J. (2012). Information packet: Post traumatic stress disorder and children in foster care. Retrieved from http://www.nrcpfc.org/is/downloads/info_packets/pts.

Heltzer, J.E., Robins, L.N., & McEvoy, L. (1987). Posttraumatic stress disorder in the general population. *New England Journal of Medicine, 317,* 1630-1634.

Hemingway, E. (1957). *A farewell to arms.* New York, NY: Scribner.

Hodas, G.R. (2006). *Responding to childhood trauma: The promise and practice of trauma informed care.* Pennsylvania Office of Mental Health and Substance Abuse Services.

Hodgetts, S., Zwaigenbaum, L., & Nicholas, D. (2015). Profile and predictors of service needs for families of children with autism spectrum disorders. *Autism, 19*(6), 673-683.

Hoge, C.W., Castro, C.A., Messer, S.C., McGurk, D., Cutting, D.I., & Koffman, R.L. (2004). Combat duty in Iraq and Afghanistan, mental health problems and barriers to care. *New England Journal of Medicine. 251,* 13-19.

Hoge, E.A., Austin, E.D., & Pollack, M.H., (2007). Resilience: Research evidence for conceptual considerations for posttraumatic stress disorder. *Depression and Anxiety, 24*(2), 139-152.

Hoge, M.A., Morris, J.A., Daniels, A.S., Stuart, G.W., Huey, L.Y., & Adams, N. (2007). An action plan for behavioral health workforce development: A framework for discussion. Rockville, MD: Substance Abuse and Mental Health Services Administration.

Hollins, S., & Kloeppel, D.A. (1989). Double handicap: Mental retardation and death in the family. *Death Studies, 13,* 31-38.

Hong, C., & Lee. I. (2012). Effects of neurofeedback training on attention in children with intellectual disability. *Journal of Neurotherapy, 16*(2), 110-122.

Horowitz, M.J., Siegel, B., Holen, A., Bonnano, G.A., Milbrath, C., & Stinson, C.H. (1997). Diagnostic disorder for complicated grief disorder. *American Journal of Psychiatry, 154*, 904-910

Howard, S., & Crandall, M.W. (2007). Post Traumatic Stress Disorder, *Washington Academy of Sciences, 93*(4), 1.

Hurley, A.D., Tomasulo, D.J., & Pfadt, A.G. (1998). Individual and group psychotherapy approaches for person with mental retardation and developmental disabilities. *Journal of Developmental and Physical Disabilities, 10*(4), 365-386.

Hyman, S.M., Gold, S.N., & Cott, M.A., (2003). Forms of social support that moderate PTSD in childhood sexual abuse survivors. *Journal of Family Violence, 18*, 295-300.

Ippen, C.G., Ford, J., Racusin, R., Acker, M., Bosquet, M., Rogers, K.,...Edwards, J. (2002). *Traumatic Events Screening Inventory – Parent Report Revised.* Retrieved from https://www.ptsd.va.gov.

Iwata, B., & Dozier, C.L. (2008). Clinical application of functional analysis methodology. *Behavior Analysis in Practice, 1*(1), 3-9.

Jacobs, S., & Prigerson, H. (2000). Psychotherapy of traumatic grief: a review of evidence for psychotherapeutic treatments. *Death Studies, 24*, 479-96.

Jahoda, M. (1977). *Freud and the dilemma of psychology.* London: Hogarth Press.

Jakupcak, M., Conybeare, D., Phelps, L., Hunt, S., Holmes, H., Felker, B.,...McFall, M.E. (2007). Anger, hostility, and aggression among Iraq and Afghanistan war veterans reporting PTSD and subthreshold PTSD. *Journal of Traumatic Stress, 2*(6), 945-954.

James, B. (1989). *Treating traumatized children.* New York, NY: The Free Press.

Jennings, A. (2004). *The damaging consequences of violence and trauma: Facts, discussion points, and recommendations for the behavioral health system.* Alexandra, VA: National Association of State Mental Health Program Directors, National Technical Assistance Center for State Mental Health Planning.

Joyce, T., Globe, A., & Moody, C. (2006). Assessment of the component skills for cognitive therapy in adults with intellectual disability. *Journal of Applied Research in Intellectual Disabilities, 19*, 17-23.

Kabat-Zinn, J., Massion, A.O., Kristeller, J., & Peterson, L.G. (1992). Effectiveness of a meditation-based stress reduction program in the treatment of anxiety disorders. *American Journal of Psychiatry, 149*, 936-943.

Keller, A., Lhewa, D., Rosenfeld, B., Sachs, E., Aladjem, A., Cohen, I.,...Porterfield, K. (2006). Traumatic experiences and psychological distress in an urban refugee population seeking treatment services. *Journal of Nervous and Mental Disease, 194*, 188-194.

Kemp, K., Signal, T., Bostros, H., Taylor, N., & Prentice, K. (2014). Equine facilitated therapy with children and adolescents who have been sexually abused: A program evaluation study. *Journal Child Family Studies, 23*, 558-566.

Kendall-Tackett, K. (2002). The health effects of childhood abuse: Four pathways by which abuse can influence health. *Child Abuse Neglect, 26*(6-7), 715-729.

Kessler, R.C., Sonnega, A., Bromet, E., Hughes, M., & Nelson, C.B. (1995). Posttraumatic stress disorder in the National Comorbidity Study. *Archives of General Psychiatry, 52*, 1048-1060.

Kilcommons, A., & Morrison, A.P. (2005). Relationships between trauma and psychosis: An exploration of cognitive and dissociative factors. *Acta Psychiatrica Scandinavica, 112*(5), 351-359.

Kimerling, R., Ouimette, P., & Wolfe, J. (2002). *Gender and PTSD.* New York, NY: The Guildford Press.

Kinnealey, M., Koenig, K.P., & Smith, S. (2011), Relationships between sensory modulation and social supports and health-related quality of life. *American Journal of Occupational Therapy, 65*(3), 320-327.

Knapp, L.G., Barrett, R.P., Groden, G., & Groden, J. (1992). The nature and prevalence of fears in developmentally disabled children and adolescents: A preliminary investigation. *Journal of Developmental and Physical Disabilities, 4*(3), 195-203.

Kolko, D.J., Hurlburt, M.S., Jinjin, Z., Barth, R.P., Leslie, L.K., & Burns, B.J. (2010). Posttraumatic stress symptoms in children and adolescents referred for child welfare investigation. *Child Maltreatment, 15*(1), 48-63.

Kung, S., Espinel, A., Lapid, M.I. (2012). A treatment of nightmares with Prazosin: A systematic review. *Mayo Clinic Proceedings, 87*(9), 890-900.

Lauterbach, D., Rajvee, V., & Rakow, M. (2005). The relationship between posttraumatic stress disorder and self-reported health problems. *Psychosomatic Medicine, 67*(6), 939-947.

LeBel, J., Champagne, T., Stromberg, N., & Coyle, R. (2010). Integrating sensory and trauma-informed interventions: A Massachusetts state initiative, part 1. *Mental Health Special Interest Quarterly, 33*(1), 1-4.

Lee, J.S., Lee, M.S., Lee, J.Y., Cornelissen, G., Otsuka, K., & Halberg, F. (2003). Effects of diaphragmatic breathing on ambulatory blood pressure and heart rate. *Biomedicine and Pharmacotherapy, 57,* 87-91.

Lemmon, V.A., & Mizes, J.S. (2002). Effectiveness of exposure therapy: a study of posttraumatic stress disorder and mental retardation. *Cognitive and Behavioral Practice, 4,* 317-23.

Levitas, A.S., & Gibson, S.F. (2001). Predictable crises in the lives of people with mental retardation. *Mental Health Aspects of Developmental Disabilities. 3,* 89-100.

Levy, T.M. (1999). *Handbook of attachment interventions.* Cambridge, MA: Academic Press.

Lew, M., Matta, C., Tripp-Tebo, C., & Watts, D. (2006). Dialectical behavior therapy for individuals with intellectual disabilities: A program description. *Mental Health Aspects of Developmental Disabilities, 9*(1), 1-13.

Libby, D.J., Reddy, F., Pilver, D., & Desai, R. (2012). The use of yoga in specialized VA PTSD treatment programs. *International Journal of Yoga Therapy, 22,* 79-87.

Lindley, S.E., Carlson, E., & Sheikh, J. (2000). Psychotic symptoms in posttraumatic stress disorder. *CNS Spectrums,* Sept; 5(9): 52-57.

Linehan, M. (1993). *Cognitive behavioral treatment of borderline personality disorder.* New York, NY: Guilford Press.

Lutz, A., Greischar, L.L., Rawlings, N.B., Ricard, M., & Davidson, R.J. (2004). Long term meditators self-induce high-amplitude gamma synchrony during mental practice. *Proceedings of the National Academy of Sciences, 101*(46), 16369-16373.

Lynch, T.R., Trost, W.T., Salsmann, N., & Linehan, M.M. (2007). Dialectical behavior therapy for borderline personality disorder. *Annual Review of Clinical Psychology. 3,* 181-205.

Macklin, M.L., Metzger, L.J., Litz, B.T., McNally, R.J., Lasko, N.B., Orr, S.P., & Pitman, R.K. (1998). Lower pre-combat intelligence is a risk factor for posttraumatic stress disorder. *Journal of Consulting and Clinical Psychology, 2,* 323-326.

Malcolm, D., & Hiebert, B. (1986). Cognitive stress-inoculation training for anger outbursts with a 30-year-old mentally retarded residential patient: A case study. *Journal of Special Education, 10,* 139-145.

Marich, J. (2014). *Trauma made simple: Competencies in assessment treatment and working with survivors.* Eau Claire, WI: PESI Publishing and Media, Inc.

Marshall, R.D., Beebe, K.L., Oldham, M., & Zaninelli, R. (2001). Efficacy and safety of paroxetine treatment for chronic PTSD: A fixed-dose, placebo-controlled study. *American Journal of Psychiatry, 158,* 1982-1988.

Martorell, A., & Tsakanikos, E. (2008). Traumatic experiences and life events in people with intellectual disability. *Current Opinion in Psychiatry, 5,* 445-448.

Matich-Maroney, J. (2003). Mental health implications for sexually abused adults with mental retardation: Some clinical research findings. *Mental Health Aspects of Developmental Disabilities, 6*(1), 11-20.

Matsakis, A. (1994). *Post-traumatic stress disorder: A clinician's guide: A complete treatment guide.* Oakland, CA: New Harbinger.

Matson, J.L. & Bamburg, J.W. (1998). Reliability of the assessment of dual diagnoses (ADD). *Research in Developmental Disabilities, 19*(1), 89-95.

Matson, J.L., Gardner, W.I., Coe, D.A., & Sovner, R. (1991). A scale for evaluating emotional disorders in severely and profoundly mentally retarded persons. *British Journal of Psychiatry, 159,* 404-409.

Mazefsky, C.A., Pelphrey, K.A., & Dahl, R.E. (2012). The need for a broader approach to emotional regulation research in autism. *Child Development Perspectives, 6*(1), 92-97.

McCarthy, J. (2001). Post-traumatic stress disorder in people with learning disability. *Advances in Psychiatric Treatment, 7,* 163-169.

McClure, K.S., Halpern, J., Wolper, P.A., Donahue, J.J. (2009). Emotion regulation and intellectual disability. *Journal on Developmental Disabilities, 15,* 38-44.

McCreary, B.D., & Thompson, J. (1999). Psychiatric aspects of sexual abuse involving persons with developmental disabilities. *The Canadian Journal of Psychiatry, 44,* 350-355.

McEwen, B.S. (2005). Stressed or stressed out: What is the difference? *Journal of Psychiatry and Neuroscience, 30,* 315-318.

McNally, R.J., & Shin L.M. (1995). Association of intelligence with severity of posttraumatic stress disorder in Vietnam combat veterans. *The American Journal of Psychiatry, 6,* 936-8.

Meichenbaum, D. (1975). Self-instructional methods. In F.H., Kanfer & A.P. Goldstein (Eds.). *Helping people change.* (pp. 357-391). New York, NY: Pergamon Press.

Meisel, V., Servera, M., Garcia-Banda, G., Cardo, E., & Moreno, I. (2013). Neurofeedback and standardized pharmacological intervention in ADHD: A randomized controlled trial with six-month follow up. *Biological Psychology, 94*(1), 12-21.

Menolascino, F. (1977). Challenges in mental retardation. *Progressive ideologies and services,* (pp. 126-127). New York, NY: Human Science Press.

Merra. T. (2005). *Dialectical behavior therapy in private practice: A practical and comprehensive guide.* Oakland, CA: New Harbinger Publications, Inc.

Mevissen, L., & de Jongh, A. (2010). PTSD and its treatment in people with intellectual disabilities: A review of the literature. *Clinical Psychology Review, 30*(3), 308-316.

Mevissen, L., Lievegoed, and de Jongh, A. (2011). EMDR treatment with people with mild intellectual disabilities and PTSD: 4 Cases. *Psychiatric Quarterly, 82*(1), 43-57.

Miller, R. (2009). *Yoga Nidra integrative restoration.* (PowerPoint presentation). Retrieved June 2, 2009, from iayt.fmdrl.org/index.cfm?event=c.getAttachment&ridd+2013

Mills, K.L., Teesson, M., Ross, J., & Peters, L. (2006). Trauma, PTSD, and substance use disorders: findings from the Australian National Survey of Mental Health and Well-Being. *American Journal of Psychiatry, 163*(4), 652-658.

Moreira, P., Santos, S., Padrao, P., Cordeiro, T., Bessa, M., Valente, H.,...Moreira, A. (2010). Food patterns according to sociodemographics, physical activity, sleeping and obesity in Portuguese children. *International Journal of Environmental Research and Public Health, 7,* 1121-1138.

Morey, R., Gold, A.L., & McCarthy, G. (2012). Amygdala volume changes with posttraumatic stress disorder in a large case-controlled veteran group. *Archives of General Psychiatry, 69*(11), 1169-1178.

Moss, S., Patel, P., Prosser, H., Goldberg, D., Simpson, N., Rowe, S., & Lucchino, R. (1993). Psychiatric morbidity in older people with moderate and severe learning disability. 1: Developmental and reliability of the patient Interview (PAS-ADD). *British Journal of Psychiatry, 163,* 471-480.

Mylle, J., & Maes, M. (2004). Partial posttraumatic stress disorder revisited. *Journal of Affective Disorders, 78*(1), 37-48.

Napoletan, A. (2013). *Caregiver PTSD: Fact or fiction.* Retrieved from http://alzjourney.com National Down Syndrome Society. (n.d.). Obstructive sleep apnea and Down syndrome. Retrieved March 10, 2018 from https://ndss.org

Nevins, R., Finch, S., Hickling, E.J., & Barnett, S.D., (2013). The Saratoga War Horse Project: A case study of the treatment of psychological distress in a veteran of Operation Iraqi Freedom. *Advances in Mind Body Medicine, 27*(4), 22-25.

Newton, R. (2014). *Exploring the experiences of living with psychiatric service dogs for veterans with posttraumatic stress disorder* (master's thesis). Adler School of Professional Psychology, Chicago, IL.

Nezu, C.M., Nezu, A.M., & Arean, P. (1991). Assertiveness and problem-solving training for mildly mentally retarded persons with dual diagnoses. *Research in Developmental Disabilities, 12*(4), 371-386.

Novak, T., Scanlan, J.N., McCaul, D., MacDonald, N., & Clarke, T. (2012). Pilot study of a sensory room in an acute inpatient psychiatric unit. *Australian Psychiatry, 20*(5), 401-406.

Novembre, G., Zanon, M., & Silani, G. (2014). Empathy for social exclusion involves the sensory-discriminative component of pain: A within-subject fMRI study. *Social Cognitive and Affective Neuroscience,10*(2), 153-164.

Oathamshaw, S.C., & Haddock, G. (2006). Do people with intellectual disabilities and psychosis have the cognitive skills required to undertake • Cognitive Behavioral Therapycognitive behavioral therapy? *Journal of Applied Research in Intellectual Disabilities, 19*(1), 35-46.

Oconghaile, A., & DeLisi, L.E. (2015). Distinguishing schizophrenia from posttraumatic stress disorder with psychosis. *Current Opinion in Psychiatry, 28*(3), 249-255.

Ochsner, K.N., Ray, R.D., Cooper J.C., Robertson, E.R., Chopra, S., Gabrieli, J.D., & Gross, J.J. (2004). For better or worse: Neural system supporting the cognitive down-and-up-regulation of negative emotion. *Neuroimage, 23* (2), 483-499.

O'Haire, M.E. (2013). Animal-assisted intervention for autism spectrum disorder: A systematic literature review. *Journal Autism and Developmental Disorders, 43*(7), 1606-1622.

O'Haire, M.E., Guerin, N.A., & Kirkham, A.C. (2015). Animal-assisted intervention for trauma: A systematic literature review. *Frontiers in Psychology, 7*(6), 1121.

O'Hare, M.W., Ghoneim, M.M., Hinrichs, J.V., Mehta, M.P., & Wright, E.J. (1989). Psychological consequences of surgery: Psychological preparation of mothers of preschool children. *Psychosomatic Medicine, 51,* 356-370.

Ozer, E., & Weiss, D. (2004). Who develops posttraumatic stress disorder? *Current Directions in Psychological Science, 13*(4), 169-172.

Park, C.L., & Adler, N.E. (2003). Coping style as a predictor of health and well-being across the first year of medical school. *Health Psychology, 22*(6), 627-31.

Pecora, P.J., Kessler, R.C., Williams, J., O'Brien, K., Downs, A.C., English, D. & Holmes, K. (2005). Improving family foster care: Findings from the Northwest Foster Care Alumni Study. Retrieved from: http://www.casey.org/resources/publications/pdf/improvingfamilyfostercare_fr.pdf.

Peuhkuri, K., Sihvola, N., & Korpela, R. (2012). Diet promotes sleep duration and quality. *Nutrition Research, 32,* 309-319.

Perkonigg, A., Kessler, R.C., Storz., & Wittchen, H.U. (2000). Traumatic events and post- traumatic stress disorder in the community: Prevalence, risk factors and comorbidity. *Acta Psychiatric Scandinavica, 101*(1), 46-59.

Pert, C., Jahoda, A., & Stenfert, K. B. (2013). • Cognitive Behavioral Therapy- Cognitive behavioral therapy from the perspective of clients with mild intellectual disabilities: a qualitative investigation of process issues. *Journal of Intellectual Disability Research, 57*(4), 359-369.

Pietrzak, R.H., Goldstein, R.B., Southwick, S.M., & Grant, B.F. (2011). Prevalence and axis I co-morbidity of full and partial posttraumatic stress disorder in the United States: Results from wave 2 of the national epidemiologic survey on alcohol and related conditions. *Journal of Anxiety Disorders, 25*(3), 456-465.

Pines, A., & Aronson, E. (1988). *Career burnout: Causes and cures.* New York, NY: The Free Press.

Pollack, N. (2010). Warriors at peace. *Yoga Journal, 230,* 74-77.

Pynoos, R.S., Frederick, C., Nade, R.K., Arroyo, W., & Steinberg, A. (1987). Life threat and posttraumatic stress in school-age children. *Archives of General Psychiatry. 44,* 1057-63.

Rando, T.A. (1993). *Treatment of complicated mourning.* Champaign, Illinois: Research Press.

Raphael, B. (1983). *The anatomy of bereavement.* New York, NY: Basic Books.

Razza, N.J. (1997). The challenge of treating person with posttraumatic stress disorder. *The Habilitative Mental Healthcare Newsletter, 16,* 94-98.

Razza, N.J., & Tomasulo, D.J. (2005). *Healing Trauma: The power of group treatment for people with intellectual disabilities.* Washington, D.C.: American Psychological Association.

Reiss, S., & Trenn, E. (1984). Consumer demand for outpatient mental health services for people with mental retardation. *Mental Retardation, 22*(3), 112-116.

Resick, P.A., (2001) *Clinical Psychology; A modular course.* Philadelphia: Taylor and Francis Group.

Resick, P.A., & Schnicke, M.K. (1993). *Cognitive processing therapy for rape victims: A treatment manual.* Thousand Oaks, CA: Sage Publications.

Resnick, H.S., Falsetti, S.A., Kilpatrick, D.G., & Freedy, J.R., (1996). Assessment of rape and other civilian trauma-related post-traumatic stress disorder: Emphasis on assessment of potentially traumatic events. In T.W. Miller (Ed.), Theory and assessment of *stressful life events* (pp. 235- 2716). Madison, CT: International University Press.

Ritchie, E. (2002). Psychiaty in the Korean War: Perils, PIES, and prisoners of war. *Military Medication, 167*(11): 898-903.

Rosenberg, S.D., Mueser, K.T., Friedman, M.J., Gorman, P.G., Drake, R.E., Vidaver, R.M., & Jankowski, M.K. (2001). Developing effective treatments for posttraumatic disorders among people with severe mental illness. *Psychiatric Services, 52,* 1453-1461.

Rosenbloom, D., & Williams, M.B. (1999). *Life after trauma: A workbook for healing.* New York, NY: The Guilford Press.

Rosenthal, J.Z., Grosswald, S., Ross, R., & Rosenthal, N. (2011). Effects of Transcendental Meditation in veterans of Operation Enduring Freedom and Operation Iraqi Freedom with posttraumatic stress disorder: a pilot study. *Military Medicine, 176*(6), 626-630.

Rueda, M.R., Pax-Alonso, P.M. (2013). Executive function and emotional development. *Encyclopedia on early childhood development.* Universidad de Granada, Spin, Basque Center on Cognition, Brain, and Language, Spain.

Russell, A., & Shab, B. (2003). Posttraumatic stress disorder and abuse. *Developmental Disabilities Digest, 30*(2), 1-8.

Ryan, R. (1994). Post-traumatic stress disorder in persons with developmental disabilities. *Community Mental Health Journal, 30,* 45-53.

Samson, A.C., Huber, O., & Gross, J.J. (2012). Emotional reactivity and regulation in adults with autism spectrum disorders. *Emotion, 12*(4), 659-665.

Samson, A.C., Phillips, J.M., Parker, Karen, K.J., Shah, S., Gross, J.J., & Hardan, A.Y. (2013). Emotional dysregulation and the core features of autism spectrum disorder. *Journal Autism Developmental Disorders, 44*(7), 1766-1772.

Sareen, J., Cox, B., Goodwin, R., & Asmundson, G. (2005). Co-occurrence of post-traumatic stress disorder with positive psychotic symptoms in a nationally representative sample. *Journal of Traumatic Stress, 18*(4), 313-322.

Schiraldi, G.R. (2000). *The post-traumatic stress disorder sourcebook: A guide to healing, recovery, and growth.* Los Angeles, CA: Lowell House.

Schnurr, P.P., Vielhauer, M.J., & Weathers, F.W. (1995). *Brief Trauma Interview.* Unpublished interview.

Schottenbauer, M.A., Glass, C.R., Arnkoff, D.B., & Gray, S.H. (2008). Contributions of psychodynamic approaches to treatment of PTSD and trauma: A review of the empirical treatment and psychopathology literature. *Psychiatry, 71*(1), 13-34.

Segal, Z.V., Williams, J.M.G., & Teasdale, J.D. (2002). *Mindfulness-based cognitive therapy for depression: A new approach to preventing relapse.* New York, NY: Guilford Press.

Seidler, G.H., & Wagner, F.E. (2006). Comparing the efficacy of EMDR and trauma-focused cognitive-behavioral therapy in the treatment of PTSD: A meta-analytic study. *Psychological Medicine, 36*(11), 1515-1522.

Selby, J. (1999). *Traumatic grief: Diagnosis, treatment, and prevention.* East Sussex, United Kingdom: Psychology Press.

Seltzer, M.M., Almeida, D.M., Greenberg, J.S., Savla, J., Stawski, R.S, Hong, J., & Taylor, J.L. (2009). Psychosocial and biological markers of daily lives in midlife parents of children with disabilities. *Journal of Health and Social Behavior, 50*(1), 1-5.

Serpell, J.A., (2010). Animal-assisted interventions in historical perspective. In A.H. Fine (Ed.), *Handbook on animal-assisted therapy: Theoretical foundations and guidelines for practice* (pp. 17-32). San Diego, CA: Academic Press.

Serpell, J.A., Coppinger, R., & Fine, A.H. (2000). The welfare of assistance and therapy animals: An ethical comment. In A.H. Fine (Ed.). *Handbook of animal-assisted therapy: Theoretical foundations and guidelines for practice* (pp. 415-431). London: Academic Press.

Shapiro, F. (1989). Efficacy of the eye moment desensitization procedure in the treatment of traumatic memories. *Journal of Traumatic Stress, 2,* 199-223.

Shapiro, F. (2001). *Eye Movement Desensitization and Reprocessing: Basic principles, protocols, and procedures.* (2nd ed.). New York, NY: The Guilford Press.

Singh, N.N., Lancioni, G.E., Winton, A.S.W., Adkins, A.D., Singh, J., & Ashvind, N. (2007). Mindfulness training assists individuals with moderate mental retardation to maintain their community placements. *Behavior Modification, 31*(6), 800-814.

Skoff, B. (2004). Executive functions in developmental disabilities. *Insights on Learning Disabilities, 15*(2), 1-10.

Snow, D.L., Swan, S.C., Raghavan, C., Connell, C.M., & Kelin, I. (2003). The relationship of work stressors, coping, and social support to psychological symptoms among female secretarial employees. *Work and Stress, 17,* 241-63.

Sobsey, D. (1994). *Violence in the lives of people with disabilities: The end of silent acceptance.* Baltimore, MD: P.H. Brooks.

Sorensen, M. (2015). The neurology of music for post-traumatic stress disorder treatment: A theoretical approach for social work implications. *Master of Social Work Clinical Research Papers.* 528. https://sophia.stkate.edu/msw_papers/528.

Souter, M.A., & Miller, M.D. (2007). Do animal-assisted activities effectively treat depression? A meta-analysis. *Anthrozoos, 20*(2), 167-180.

Sprague, C. (2008). Judges and child trauma: Findings form the National Child Traumatic Stress Network/National Council of Juvenile and Family Court Judges Focus Groups. *NCTSN Service Systems Brief, 2*(2). Los Angeles, CA: National Center for Traumatic Stress.

Sroufe, L.A. (1979). The coherence of individual development. *American Psychologist, 34*(10), 834-841.

Stanley, J.A., Muramatsu, N., Heller, T., Hughes, S., Johnson, T.P, & Ramirez-Valles, J. (2010). *Journal of Intellectual Disabilities Research, 54*(8), 749-761.

Stovall-McClough, K.C., & Cloitre, M. (2006). Unresolved attachment, PTSD, and dissociation in women with childhood abuse histories. *Journal of Consulting and Clinical Psychology, 74*, 219- 228.

Strakowski, S.M., Keck, P.E. Jr., McElroy, S.L., Lonczak, H.S., & West, S.A. (1995). Chronology of comorbid and principal syndromes in first-episode psychosis. *Comprehensive Psychiatry, 36*(2), 106-112.

Substance Abuse and Mental Health Services Administration (2014). *SAMHSA's concept of trauma and guidance for a trauma-informed approach.* HHS Publication No. (SMA) 14-4884. Rockville, MD: Substance Abuse and Mental Health Administration.

Sullivan, P. (2009). Violence exposure among children with disabilities. *Clinical Child and Family Psychology Review, 12*(2) 196-216.

Sullivan, P.M., & Knutson, J.F. (2000). Maltreatment and disabilities: A population based epidemiological study. *Child Abuse and Neglect, 24*, 1257-1273.

Surmeli, T., & Ertem, A. (2007). EEG neurofeedback treatment of patients with Down Syndrome. *Journal of Neurotherapy, 11*(1), 63-68.

Tharner, G. (2006). About the application of EMDR in the treatment of people with a mild intellectual disability. In Robert, D. (Ed.), *Perspectief. Gedragsproblemen, psychiatrische stoornissen en lichte verstandelijke,* Bohn, Stafleu ven Loghum, pp. 145-168.

Tomasulo, D.J., & Razza, N.J. (2007). Posttraumatic stress disorders. In R. Fletcher, E. Loschen, C. Stavrakaki, & M. First (Eds.), *Diagnostic manual – intellectual disability (DM- ID): A textbook of diagnosis of mental disorders in persons with intellectual Disability* (pp. 365- 378). Kingston, NY: National Association for the Dually Diagnosed.

Tottenham, N., Hare, T.A., & Casey, B.J. (2011). Behavioral assessment of emotion discrimination, emotional regulation, and cognitive control in childhood, adolescence, and adulthood. *Frontiers in Psychology, 2*(39).

Tugate, M.M., & Fredrickson, B.L. (2004). Resilient individuals use positive emotions to bounce back from negative emotional experiences. *Journal of Personality and Social Psychology, 86*(2), 320-333.

Tyrer, F., McGrother, C.W., Thorp, C.F., Donaldson, M., Bhaumik, S., Watson, J.M., & Hollin, C. (2006). Physical aggression towards others in adults with learning disabilities: Prevalence and associated factors. *Journal of Disabilities Research, 50,* 295-304.

Uma, K., Nagendra, H.R., Nagarathna, R., Vaidehi, S., & Seethalakshmi, R. (1989). *Journal Mental Deficiency Research, 33,* 415 – 21.

United Cerebral Palsy and Children's Rights. (2006). A case for action for children and youth with disabilities in foster care. Retrieved November 12, 2016, from http://www.ucp.org/uploads/Forgotten ChildrenFINAL.pdf

Unwin, G., Tsimopoulou, I., Stenfert, K., & Asmi, S. (2016). Effectiveness of • Cognitive Behavioral Therapycognitive behavioral therapy (CBT) programs for anxiety or depression in adults with intellectual disabilities: A review of the literature. *Research in Developmental Disabilities, 51-52,* 60-75.

Valenti-Hein, D., & Schwartz, L. D. (1995). *The sexual abuse interview for those with developmental disabilities.* Santa Barbara, CA: James Stanfield Company.

van der Kolk, B.A., (1996). The complexity of adaptation to trauma: Self-regulation, stimulus discrimination, and characterological development. In B.A. van der Kolk, A.C. MacFarlane, & L. Weisaeth (Eds.), *Traumatic stress: The effects of overwhelming experience on mind, body, and society* (pp. 182-213). New York, NY: Guildford Press.

van der Kolk, B.A. (2006). Clinical implications of neuroscience research in PTSD. *Annals of the New York Academy of Sciences, 1071*, 277-293.

van der Kolk, B.A., Hodgdon, H., Gapen, M., Musicaro, R., Suvak, M.K., Hamlin E., & Spinazzola, J. (2016). A randomized controlled study of neurofeedback for chronic PTSD. *PLOS One, 11*(12). https://doi:10.1371/journal.pone.0166752

Veronen, L.J., & Kilpatrick, D.G. (1982). *Stress inoculation training for victims of rape: Efficacy and differential findings*. Symposium conducted at the 16th Annual Convention of the Association for the Advancement of Behavior Therapy, Los Angeles.

Vig, S., Chinitz, S., & Shulman, L. (2005). Young children in foster care – Multiple vulnerabilities and complex service needs. *Infants and Young Children, 18*(2), 147-160.

Wadsworth, J., & Harper, D.C. (1991). Grief and bereavement in mental retardation: A need for a new understanding. *Death Studies, 15*, (3), 281-292.

Weathers, F.W., Blake, D.D., Schnurr, P.P., Kaloupek, D.G., Marx, B.P., & Keane, T.M. (2013). The Clinician –Administered PTSD Scale for DSM-5 (CAPS-5). National Center for PTSD. Retrieved from http://www.ptsd.va.gov

Weiss, D. S., & Marmar, C.R. (1996). The Impact of Event Scale-Revised. In J.P. Wilson & T.M. Keane (Eds.), *Assessing psychological trauma and PTSD* (pp. 399-411). New York, NY: Guilford Press.

Whitman. T.L. (1990). Self-regulation and mental retardation. *American Journal on Mental Retardation, 94*(4), 347-362.

Wieland, J., Warenaar, K.J., Dautovic, E., & Zitman, F.G. (2013). Characteristics of posttraumatic stress disorder in patients with an intellectual disability. *European Psychiatrist, 28*(1), 1.

Wigham, S., Taylor, J. & Hatton, C. (2014). A prospective study of the relationship between adverse life events and trauma in adults with mild to moderate intellectual disabilities. *Journal of Intellectual Disability Research, 58*(12), 1131-1140.

Wilgosh, L. (1993). Sexual abuse of children with disabilities: Intervention and treatment issues for parents. *Developmental Disabilities Bulletin, 21*(2), 1-12.

Williams, M.B., & Poijula, S. (2002). *The PTSD workbook: Simple, effective techniques for overcoming traumatic stress symptoms*. Oakland, California: New Harbinger Publications.

Wilson, J.P. (1994). The historical evolution of PTSD diagnostic criteria: from Freud to DSM-IV. *Journal of Traumatic Stress. 7*(4), 681-698.

Wimer, B. (2017). *Sensory techniques for trauma, self-harm, and dysregulation*. Eau Claire, Wisconsin: PESI, Inc.

Wood, L., Giles-Corti, B., & Bulsara, M. (2005). The pet connection: Pets as a conduit for social capital? *Social Sciences and Medicine, 61*(6), 1159-1173.

Index

A

ACEs viii, 8, 125-126, 131, 141, 145, 152
Aggression vii, 11, 13, 18, 24, 31, 33-35, 37-38, 53-54, 60, 62, 65-66, 71, 93, 95, 108, 117-118, 120, 128-130, 133, 135-136, 139-141, 163, 170
Anger outbursts vii, 18, 71, 88, 93, 101, 106, 115, 142, 165
Animal assisted interventions 106
Antidepressants 20, 107, 115, 138, 142, 146
Assertiveness training vii, 94, 106
Assessment of Dual Diagnosis (ADD) 45, 165
Assessment measures vi, xi, 44-46
Autism 21-22, 54, 70, 96, 102, 106, 120, 125, 139, 141-145, 147
Avoidance behaviors vi, 30-31, 35, 44, 53, 67-68, 100, 127

B

Behavioral symptoms 29, 34, 72
Boundaries 58-59, 61-62, 65-66, 87-88, 110-111, 118, 153-154
Burnout vi, 70-72, 167

C

Case studies viii, xii, 88-89, 91-92, 96-97, 123, 128
Childhood abuse 8, 34, 170
Co-morbidity vi, 38, 41

D

Developmental trauma v, 23-24
Diagnostic Assessment for the Severely Handicapped (DASH-II) 45
Dialectical Behavior Therapy vii, 89, 94-95, 159-160, 164-165
DM-ID 30-31
DM-ID-2 30-32
DSM-I 26
DSM-II 26
DSM-III 26-27
DSM-III-R 27
DSM-IV 28, 47, 171
DSM-IV-TR 28-29
DSM-5 25, 29-31, 36, 38, 40, 43-45, 47, 158, 171

E

Emotional dysregulation v, 20-22, 24, 94, 103
Emotional regulation skills v, vii, 21-23, 102-104
Executive functioning deficits 22
Exposure Therapy vii, 88, 99-100, 164
Eye Movement Desensitization Reprocessing vii, 88-92

F

Family environment vii, 122

G

Glasgow Anxiety Scale for People with Intellectual Disabilities (GAS-ID) 45, 160

H

Hebbian theory 83-84
Historical references to PTSD v, 25

I

Impact of Event Scale – Intellectual Disabilities (IES-IDs) 45, 162

M

Medical trauma vii, 119, 157, 162
Meditation vii, 95-98, 104, 157, 160, 163, 168
Mindfulness vii, 94-96, 104, 169
Music Therapy vii, 104, 107

N

Neurofeedback vii, 89, 97-98, 160, 162, 165, 170-171
Neuroplasticity vii, 83

P

Peri-traumatic factors vi, 79
Pharmacological interventions vii, 107-108, 165

Post-traumatic factors vi, 78-79
Predictor variables for PTSD vii, 80
Pre-traumatic factors vi, 78
Psychiatric Assessment Schedule for Adults with Developmental Disabilities Checklist (PAS-ADD-10) 46, 166
Psychodynamic Psychotherapy vii, 97
Psychosis vi, 31, 40-42, 158-159, 164, 166-167, 170
Psychotropic medications v, viii, 15, 34, 49, 52, 102, 107-108, 115, 119, 126, 132, 139, 141-142, 146, 151
PTSD in children vi, 162
PTSD in Children vi, 46, 162

Q

Questionnaires xi, 44-48, 50-51, 123, 127

R

Relaxation Response Training vii, 99
Resiliency vi-vii, 58-59, 68, 77, 80-82, 85, 106, 149, 153
Restraints v, 6, 14, 49, 102, 139

S

Safety vii, xii, 8, 12-3, 23, 50, 52, 57-58, 60-61, 64-67, 70, 74, 83-88, 102, 105, 107-110, 116-117, 120, 132, 135-137, 152-154, 158, 165
Self-care plans vi, 71-72, 86
Sensory modulation vii, 101, 158, 164
Sexual trauma v, 8
Sleep disturbances vii, 25, 27, 34, 51, 112-113, 115, 142
Social support vii, 59, 64, 66, 72, 79-81, 112, 154, 163-164, 169
Somatic symptoms vi, 39-40
Strategies for administrators and managers 60-65
Strategies for parents vi, 67
Stress Inoculation Training vii, 88, 171
Subthreshold PTSD 36-38, 55, 106, 135, 153, 160, 163

T

Timeline of events viii, 127, 133, 142, 146, 147
Trauma induced behaviors vi
Types of trauma v, xii, 2, 7, 44, 45, 59, 62, 79, 85, 91, 153

Y

Yoga vii, 89, 98-99, 164, 166-167

www.ingramcontent.com/pod-product-compliance
Lightning Source LLC
Chambersburg PA
CBHW060420300426
44111CB00018B/2913